WASN'T EXPECTING THIS

What people are saying about *Wasn't Expecting This*

"Erma Bombeck famously found meaning in a place no one else was looking – the everyday lives of everyday women. Adina Ciment does her foremother proud with these essays of surviving school supply shopping, summer camp, movie night negotiations – and breast cancer. Her work is humorous, hopeful and human. Some bit of Erma lives in these pages."

Leonard Pitts, Jr. Pulitzer Prize-winning author of *The Last Thing You Surrender*

"Adina writes with the clarity of a teacher, the wit of a blogger and the fearlessness of a superhero because she is all three. This book will take you to the edge of what is possible for one human to endure before throwing a protective arm across your chest like a mom performing an emergency brake maneuver, reassuring you that all will be ok, even when it isn't."

Gila Pfeffer, humor and essay writer, and author of *Nearly Departed, a memoir*

"From the tremors of young womanhood and motherhood to their mortal terrors, Adina Ciment tells it all in a battle-scarred, urgent, irreverent voice, with a cool eye and a warm heart."

Tova Reich, author, most recently, of *The House of Love and Prayer: and Other Stories*

"In this often hilarious and candid memoir, Adina takes readers through the chaos of motherhood, her own battle with breast cancer, and the challenges of caring for a son with a brain tumor. Armed with a razor-sharp wit and a healthy dose of sarcasm, she navigates the absurdities of life, offering a refreshing and humorous perspective on the highs and lows of facing adversity."

Carmen Calfa, MD
Associate Professor of Clinical Medicine,
University of Miami

WASN'T EXPECTING THIS

Essays on life and family (and you know, cancer)

ADINA CIMENT

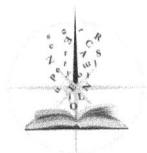

Storytellers Publishing
COLORADO, USA

Storytellers Publishing
An imprint of Journey Institute Press,
a division of 50 in 52 Journey, Inc.
journeyinstitutepress.org

Library of Congress Control Number: 2024936660
Names: Ciment, Adina
Title: Wasn't Expecting This
Description: Colorado: Storytellers Publishing, 2024
Identifiers: ISBN 979-8-9886470-2-7 (hardcover)
ISBN 978-1-964754-09-3 (paperback)
ISBN 978-1-964754-10-9 (ebook/kindle)
Subjects: BISAC:
BIOGRAPHY & AUTOBIOGRAPHY / Women |
BIOGRAPHY & AUTOBIOGRAPHY / Medical |
HEALTH & FITNESS / Diseases & Conditions / Cancer

First Edition
Printed in the United States of America

1 4 7 8 11 21 29 40 52 71

This book was typeset in Caslon Pro /
Neue Haas Grotesk Display Pro
Editing by Jessica Medberry, InkWhale Editorial LLC.
Cover design by Tamar Ciment

For Miriam, who told me to do this,
and for Avi, who showed me it was possible.

CONTENTS

CAREGIVER

NOTE FROM THE AUTHOR

The chapters in this book that reference Neil Gaiman and Amanda Palmer were written prior to any knowledge of the recent accusations of sexual assault against him. Neil Gaiman has long been a significant influence on my work and someone I deeply admired for his storytelling and creativity. His work shaped my understanding of narrative and inspired me as a writer.

It is profoundly disheartening to learn that someone I looked up to and respected could be accused of such harmful behavior. Acknowledging this reality is difficult, but it is important to listen to survivors and take their accounts seriously.

While I chose to leave these chapters in the book as they were originally written to reflect the journey of my own creative growth, I do so with a heavy heart. I believe it's essential to separate admiration for someone's work from blind idolization of the person behind it, and I hope this serves as a reminder that even those we admire are capable of deeply disappointing us.

AC
January 2025

FOREWORD

Timing, as they say, is everything.

Publishing is as much a word-of-mouth business as any these days, and Adina came to me with her idea for this book via her connection with my wife. She described the concept and provided the obligatory sample pages of the manuscript. I was intrigued because of the story of course and also the way these chapters had come together organically throughout her journey.

This was September of 2022. Three months later, Adina sent the finished rough draft.

What she didn't know was that a few weeks prior to receiving that finished manuscript, I myself had been diagnosed with prostate cancer.

I stared at the manuscript for more than a few days. Could I really do this? Could I publish a book that was by all accounts going to be about a much more serious fight with this monster than anything I was likely to endure? I was frightened. I didn't yet know exactly what lay ahead of me. All I knew was that I was scared of dying.

Since life wasn't going to stop just because I was scared, I eventually picked up the manuscript and began to read.

What I found surprised me. I expected a story about, not one but two, battles with the monster and the trials and tribulations, the emotional roller coasters, the anguish, and triumphs of battling cancer in multiple family members multiple times.

Sure, the battles were there, it's what prompted the book after all, but it was so much more than that. In fact, the beginning battle with the monster doesn't even arrive until about a quarter of the way through the book.

This is a book that goes beyond the incredible journey Adina and her family have undertaken because of the monster that is cancer. It is a book of essays about living despite the fear. Of being a parent, a mother, a woman. Of finding strength amidst the onslaught. There is a vulnerable honesty in these pages that demands we pay attention and learn the lessons. Through it all is the wit and tenacity of hope that Adina refused to let go of despite the many challenges she and her family faced. Written with humor and compassion, with grace and with power, these stories are filled with wisdom we can all take something away from, whether or not you are fighting the monster.

Don't worry, if you want the cancer story(ies) it's(they're) in here too, along with all the trials, tribulations, struggles, and exasperations you would expect from a tale such as this one. It's just that there is so much more to the story. Publishers are expected to say nice things about the books their authors write. Publishers aren't always expected to connect so personally with the book. This book is all the things a publisher wants when they're looking at manuscripts. It has an interesting plot, compelling characters, and is well written. This book, however, has something else as well. It has Adina.

Settle in as she invites you to ride along with her on her journey. Pay attention along the way for the lessons that seem somehow hidden in plain sight in the stories of everyday living. I know I benefitted from them immensely as I began a journey of my own.

As a publishing house we are incredibly proud to have joined Adina on her journey of publishing this book.

I hope you enjoy reading it as much as I did.

Michael Jenet
Publisher
Journey Institute Press

INTRODUCTION

Palm Reading

I wonder if everyone has a pivotal moment that transforms their lives into "before" and "after" timelines. I remember someone looking at my palm and telling me that the little indentations in my lifeline indicated some kind of personal trauma. These little dots interrupt the smoothness of the long ravine that divides my thumb from the other fingers in my hand, creating rivulets and trenches in what should be a straight and narrow line. Sometimes I look at that life line, see those marks, and wonder which traumas they represent. Is this the breast cancer one? Is this my son's brain tumor? And then I wonder if everyone has those marks, and when someone else sees them in their palm, do they think, "Is this the broken leg?" or "Is this the C-section?" And then I wonder if their traumas, which seem so trivial to me, are the dividing points that separate me from them. I look back at where I was before those "dots" made an appearance in my life and think about what I was concerned with. What bothered me. What I thought was important and what was not.

In 2012, I started a blog. It started as a way to get me to sit down and write every day. When I launched it, I had a solid two readers: myself and my mom. I don't even think my husband was reading it at the time. I used that space to record my day-to-day, to respond to current events, and to occasionally put out some fiction—some of my own work.

When breast cancer hit, my blog shifted. When my son was diagnosed with a brain tumor, it shifted again. Looking back at that little corner of cyberspace, I saw that transformation. I saw the indentations in my life line playing out in my writing and my observations. I saw how those small marks divided my life into the "before" and the "after." But I also saw how those once-a-week observations affected others.

The world is filled with grief tourists and trauma vampires who love to watch the suffering of others, voyeurs to pain and struggling. When I wrote about hard times and difficult days, my blog had more readers, I had more listeners, and more people suddenly related to the feelings and emotions I had thought were only mine. In looking back at those posts and the responses I received, I realized that my little blog served a larger purpose. And through those blog posts I saw how I had shifted roles, moving seamlessly between mother, patient, and caregiver, and sometimes losing the role of woman.

These essays are my signposts—the notches in my palm's lifeline—that mark moments and observations over ten years of joy, pain, struggle, and triumph. This book includes essays that were never posted publicly, kept safe in my drafts, that I had written only for myself. This collection brings together content from my blog entries and my previously unpublished work to tell the whole story.

These are the moments that are etched into my soul like the marks on my palm. Scarring me in one sense, marking me in another, but in the end, changing me permanently. Making me into who I am today.

MOTHER

When my oldest of my five kids was in pre-K, her teacher called a meeting with me to discuss the transition to kindergarten. My daughter was precocious. Responsible and smart, she was talking in full sentences before she was a year old. At the age of four, she took her education seriously and was a top reader and writer.

But the meeting wasn't about pushing her ahead. Instead, it was about having her repeat pre-K. She had missed the official cutoff date for entering kindergarten, and as the youngest in her class, the teachers felt she could use another year of emotional growth.

I was shocked. And at the age of twenty-eight, I was indignant. How could I keep my daughter back? How could I have her repeat pre-K? I worried about her socially. All her friends were moving ahead. How could I do this to her?

Years later—many years later—I looked back at that moment and realized I knew nothing about being a parent. The issues I thought were so important, so vital to my child's well-being, were really just nonsense in the grand scheme of things. My daughter's social calendar at the age of four was not going to define her life. In fact, having her repeat that year turned out to be a good choice.

Parenting is fraught with decisions and beliefs that are constantly tested and retested. It's a role that changes, that requires fluidity and backbone. It's a role that I took, and still take, seriously. The experiences we give our children, the values we impart, the messages we hope they take to heart (and the ones we hope they forget) impact their lives long after they leave our homes.

My meditations on motherhood have changed over the years; my outlook on how best to educate my children and raise them so that they will be happy, functional members of society has grown with them. I wanted them to be readers. I wanted them to love *Star Wars* and *Harry Potter*. I wanted them to make healthy choices. I wanted. I wanted. I wanted.

In the end, my role as "mother" was more facilitator than lecturer. In the end, my children grew into who they each were meant to be. In the end, I realized the most important part of being a parent—more than the back-to-school nights, the sleepovers, the gifts, and the discipline—was just being there.

And that role never ends.

Back to School, 2012

School starts this week, and so, like many other parents, I have taken the requisite school supply shopping trip. For those who have never had the experience, I envy you. Armed with lists provided by my children's school, I scoured the internet for the cheapest prices, the best sales, the most available downloadable coupons, and the store least likely to throw us out when my four-year-old inadvertently spills out boxes of paper clips and tacks.

Since I have five children, I first pillaged the supplies from last year, thinking that somewhere in the scores of folders and binders that still resided in their old backpacks, I would be able to recycle something.

But this year, the teachers must have pooled their ideas and decided to get a bit more precise. Instead of five folders, now my oldest son needed five specific folders. No paper, just plastic. Exact colors. None of the twenty-six folders I spread onto the living room floor were usable.

The search for supplies became even more daunting at the store. My eighth grader was convinced that five-subject

21

notebooks don't come in purple (the color required for her science class). My kids in third and fourth grade had to open each folder on the shelf to find the right ones: they needed some with pockets and prongs, some with only pockets, some with only prongs. My seventh grader, loaded down with four binders, rattled off the subjects they were for as she dropped each one onto our ever-growing pile: math, English, social studies, computers. Before I could question it, the binders were followed by a flurry of dividers, reinforcement stickers, reams of paper, and a pencil case.

Four binders? I remember when school supply shopping consisted of begging my mom for the Trapper Keeper with the cool plastic sliding latch. Once I had that, with a pack of dividers, pencils, erasers, and a case, I was done.

"What five subjects could you possibly need in math?" I asked.

In an attempt to remain cutting edge, teachers are hell-bent on providing their students with so much enrichment that managing and organizing the supplies has become a lesson in small business administration. Each subject requires its own unique set of supplies beyond a simple section in a notebook. I drew the line at the two USB drives required per child, but as I crossed off each item that was thrown in our cart, I found myself rethinking my mortgage and considered embracing homeschooling.

When we finally checked out, I assessed the damage and revisited everyone's lists. My eighth grader settled on a blue five-subject notebook that she will convince her teacher is really an off-shade of purple. The seventh grader practiced carrying all the binders and notebooks and decided she would need a larger backpack to carry everything from class to class. And the supplies for the two in the third and fourth grades, the rainbow of colorful folders and notebooks, fit perfectly in the 5-inch binder and two 3-inch binders they needed.

I didn't even know they made 5-inch binders.

As for the child going into pre-k, we escaped from the store with only one box of erasers and paperclips spilled out in aisle 12.

I realize that the teachers who created these supply lists have the best intentions, and I am eager to discover what the different colors will represent for the year. However, perhaps it is time for teachers to remember that a complex organizational strategy is an oxymoron. The adage "Less is more," particularly in the current economic climate, is probably something they should consider when making supply lists that could double as doorstoppers.

My son was excited about our shopping trip, though. Taking the receipt that easily could wrap around all five of my kids, he exclaimed, "Look! It's a jump rope!"

But alas, it was too long.

Waverunners

This is a pretty cool story.

At the end of the summer in 2012, I took a trip to the Florida Keys with my kids. Living in Florida usually lends itself to a lot of water sports and activities, but ironically, we don't get to the beach as much as one would think. I guess it's like how New Yorkers rarely get to the Statue of Liberty or the Empire State Building. Our big travel usually takes us north, not south. So instead of doing the Disney/Universal/Sea World thing, I made the radical decision to hang out at the beach in the Keys.

We got a beautiful house right on the water and I purchased all the requisite equipment—shovels, buckets, goggles, and snorkel gear. We drove on the Seven Mile Bridge and stopped to look for shells right off the road. But the best part by far was renting WaveRunners.

It was just me and the five kids, so I had to keep coming back to the dock to make sure everyone had a turn. Mind you, I hadn't been on a WaveRunner in a really long time, and I was terrified, to say the least. I started off with my youngest child, and I am lucky I didn't get a heart attack when we went out. I imagined him flying off the seat, slipping out of his life vest. Every time I turned, my heart dropped and I panicked. It was the longest ten minutes, and when we pulled into the dock for the next kid's turn, I told the owner that I didn't think I was going to be able to stay out for the whole hour.

But he just smiled and set my ten-year-old in front of me, and off we went. Again I was panicked, sure we would run into the boats that were a mile away. I imagined what they would say about me. "How irresponsible! What kind of mother is she?"

When I returned to the dock, my hand was numb from gripping the handles so tightly.

"You need to relax," the man said. "Just have fun. You'll be fine."

I took his advice, took a deep breath, and pulled out into the Gulf of Mexico again.

Pretty soon, I was relaxed. I let go of the fear of falling and drowning and just took off. My eleven-year-old son was with me, and I even let him drive. I started telling him what the man on the dock said to me. "Relax. Let go. You'll be fine."

It was an incredible experience, just me and my kids and the Gulf. There were dolphins and pelicans, and we took off into the sun. My son felt like James Bond. When it was my daughter's turn, she was excited that she was able to actually "drive" while her mother held on for dear life. But the best was when I returned to the dock for the last time. The hour was up and everyone had a turn. The man at the dock plucked my kids off the WaveRunner and then unceremoniously kicked it away from the dock while I was still on it. I looked at him, but he just laughed.

"Oh no!" he said. "Looks like you're drifting away. Better go take fifteen minutes to yourself and come back after."

I couldn't believe it.

I pulled out of the lagoon to the cheers of my kids and peeled out into the Gulf of Mexico. This time it was just me. No one to worry about or hold on to. I drove straight ahead, and soon the Florida shore seemed farther than the shore of Texas. I turned corkscrews and stood up, pushing the throttle as far as it would go. I couldn't believe that I had been so scared in the beginning, too paralyzed to even try to let go and enjoy. I couldn't believe that I had even thought of canceling the hour and not doing this.

It was exhilarating.

When I returned to the dock, my kids were waiting to give me high fives and congratulate me. I thanked the man at the dock, collected everyone, and went off to the pool to hang out and swim.

Those fifteen minutes were not just a simple gift. They highlighted a simple truth about fear. I wasn't doing something monumental. I mean, it's a WaveRunner, for crying out loud. But the "what ifs" and "what could happens" and the thoughts of "oh my God my husband will kill me" were crippling. I would have gotten off that machine after ten minutes, swearing there was no way I could go on.

But I didn't. And when I got those last moments to myself, it was more than me running free on the water. It was me embracing that small victory and realizing that I can conquer anything.

And man, it was awesome.

Happy Mother's Day, Mrs. Weasley!

As far as the Literary Mother of the Year awards go, Mrs. Weasley became a contender the moment she helped Harry Potter get onto Platform Nine and Three-Quarters in the first book. But her title was clinched forever in the seventh book of the series when she brandished her wand against Bellatrix Lestrange and yelled those five little words heard across the Potterverse: "Not my daughter, you bitch!"

It was a moment that spawned a Facebook group with over one hundred thousand members, as well as numerous comics and an entirely new group of loyal Mrs. Weasley fans. All of a sudden, "Mollywobbles" was a badass. A force to be reckoned with outside of the Burrow. A woman who could hold her own.

Truth is, I had known that all along.

My relationship with Mrs. Weasley has changed over the years. When I first met her, way back in 1998, she was the worried mother—always cooking, knitting some god-awful sweater, or fretting over her children and their eating habits. But Mrs. Weasley is far from any one-dimensional archetype. As a mother of seven children, she struggles with their different personalities, and her philosophy as a parent changes. She is exasperated with the twins, Fred and George, whose constant jokes and pranks set them on a path she doesn't particularly approve of nor want to endorse. She scuffles with her eldest son's choice of a fiancée and even tries to get him interested in another girl. She grieves as her son Percy takes sides against the family and alienates himself from them. But although she tries to control and guide her children, she is able to let go when she has to. In the end, though she makes her opinion heard loud and clear, she lets her children make their own choices.

As I read the books, my own children were growing up, and I found myself relating to Mrs. Weasley more and more. I noticed my kids' differences and quickly realized that what worked for one did not necessarily work for all. I suddenly started wishing for a clock that could tell me where all my children were (though hopefully not all in "Mortal Peril," as the Weasley clock so often indicated). I wished I had access to a Howler to reprimand one of my kids more effectively than an angry text message. I loved the Weasley home: The Burrow. The house is a mess, there isn't much money, and the father has strange hobbies, but there is always room for more people, there's always enough food, and everyone manages. Everyone feels at home.

It is Mrs. Weasley's strength that shines at the end of the series. By the time the seventh book came out, I had five children of my own, and I finally "got" Molly. That's why I wasn't surprised by her actions during the Battle of Hogwarts. There were times I wanted to sweep into my daughter's sixth-grade class and pull out a wand on some of those mean girls. Times I wanted to sit in my son's classroom and go "Crucio!" all over the teacher. For all her worrying and her crying, Mrs. Weasley is more than just a bundle of wizarding neuroses. More than a stereotype. Long before she bested Bellatrix, Molly Weasley was fighting for her children and her family and every person who ever sat at her table.

Mrs. Weasley's role moves from the periphery in the earlier books to a more formidable one as she becomes "Mom" to everyone. To her children, to Harry—even to characters like the ever-changing Tonks, the moody Remus Lupin, and impetuous Sirius Black. She is their comforter, their confidante, and their supporter. When necessary, she scolds children and adults alike and does not back off when anyone she loves is on the line.

And *that's* what being a mom is all about.

Stress, 2013

Stress has all sorts of negative effects on one's health and body.

I'm under a lot of stress right now. The biggies: new job, new house, new schools for my kids, car breaking down, very little money. You get the idea.

So aside from the elevated heart rate, the zero patience, and the total exhaustion, there is another side effect that no one ever talks about.

The "not caring" effect.

It's probably tied to the whole "no patience" thing, but today I kept a list of the things I absolutely did not care about because my current problems definitely trump everyone else on the entire planet's problems.

I did not care about the poor woman ahead of me in line at the pizza shop who took a full fifteen minutes to place her order and managed to ask more questions about a salad than I ever thought possible. And it's a pizza shop, lady. If you are asking for a slice without cheese or sauce, then you are asking for bread. Get out of line and go to the supermarket.

And I also did not care that the employee with the sophistication of a twelve-year-old behind the counter told me it would take fifteen minutes for my five slices and fries. This is a pizza shop. If pizza is your primary product, it should be made a bit faster. At least faster than the slice with no sauce and no cheese that came out of the oven way before my standard slices.

But I didn't care.

I didn't care about the family in the van in front of me in the middle of traffic, who had themselves depicted in stickered caricatures on the back windshield.

Who thought of that ridiculous idea? Because really? Your smiling stick-figure family and dog are clashing with your "Honor Student" bumper sticker. And your announcement that you have three alarmingly emaciated children just makes me want to ram the back of your Honda Odyssey with my falling-apart Accord.

But I didn't care.

I didn't care when the stay-at-home mom announced to the cashier at Target how exhausted she was because she had to wait in line so long. She must have a particularly difficult life if standing in a line is exhausting. And while I looked at her perfectly coiffed hair and fresh-from-the-gym yoga pants, I resisted the urge to shake my discount soda can and open it up in her exhausted face, because if waiting in line is the most tiring thing you have to do, well then, you need to do some laundry.

But I didn't care about her.

I didn't care when the barista screwed up my coffee because she was too busy flirting with the guy in front of me who looked like he could have been an actor but seemed like a bit of a creeper. And if you can't handle "One tall coffee, black," I don't think you should be working at Starbucks.

I didn't care when the Genius at the Genius Bar in the Apple Store went on Google to find the answer to my question. Really? That's what makes you a genius? Because had I known that there was this site called "Google" well, then, golly gee, I never would have made this appointment. You *are* a genius.

I didn't care when I walked into my new house, which is filled with so many boxes that I'm worried my neighbors might stage an Extreme Hoarding intervention, to find that the plumber never showed, the sinks are not working, and the roof is leaking.

I didn't care.

Stress does that.

I fell into my couch, closed my eyes, and didn't care about anything.

Until my friend called and asked me if I was thinner because "People who are stressed out tend to lose weight!"

I hung up on her. And ate a donut.

And I totally didn't care.

Stress does that.

iPads, iMacs, and iPhones

As I was tucking in my ten-year-old daughter one night, she dropped the bomb.

"Everyone in my class has an iPhone but me."

I'm sure it's true. In fact, I was surprised it took this long for her to ask. I've seen kids at dismissal playing. I knew that this was going to become an issue soon.

I also know that this is an age-old problem. I remember complaining to my mother that I was the only kid in class without a Walkman. I'm sure she complained to *her* mother that she was the only kid in her class without a transistor radio. Somewhere in history, there was some kid that complained to her mother that she was the only kid without that newfangled "wheel" thing.

But I can't simply respond with the stock "And if everyone was jumping off a bridge, would you do that too?" Because, really, my family is all over the iToys. We have iPads. We use an iMac and MacBook Pros. I upgrade my iPhone with each new release.

No. My reason for keeping the iStuff at bay for a bit longer is that I've noticed something alarming about the way kids with tech toys play.

They don't.

Sure, they play lots of games, and I also have some educational apps on my phone that my kids use. But the real "play"—the creating worlds with cardboard boxes, the building of forts in the living room, the death-defying challenge of "Lava" on a rainy day—those things are starting to disappear. It makes me wonder if kids are forgetting *how* to play. And maybe parents are forgetting how to play with their kids.

It's like that old book *If You Give a Moose a Muffin*. It starts with the phone and then quickly and easily progresses from there.

Maybe that's the real problem. It's so tempting to give a kid a game and let them play, and play, and play—while you do the dishes, or empty a closet, or write another chapter. But it's like taking a piece of the creativity that is innate in every kid and just crushing it. Instead of telling kids to find a game, to make one up, parents download it. The forts in the den become the virtual forts in Minecraft.

I have rules about the computer in our house. We keep the computer where we can see it. There are parental controls. And so, how can I hand my daughter a small device that has unlimited, unmonitored, unchecked internet access? And why would any parent want to do that?

Perhaps it's just me getting older. Maybe as I've aged, I've become that person who just wants to say, "If everyone jumped off the bridge, would you?" Maybe I'm out of touch with the current reality.

But I think I am in touch with it. And that's what worries me.

I know I will probably get my daughter an iPhone. And I know she won't be happy that it's the SE and not the latest model. But what's more important to me than keeping up with the times and accepting the new reality is that I want my kids to have a chance to create worlds of their own. To enjoy books. To recognize the difference between writing on a piece of paper and typing on a MacBook.

I want them to remember that. So when their own kids ask for whatever new top-of-the-line, I-must-have-it gadget, they will sigh, scratch their heads, and say those famous words:

"And if everyone was jumping off a bridge . . ."

Dear Teacher

Dear Teacher,

I am writing this to you because I have worked as an educator for over two decades and have been around the block, so to speak, in terms of teaching experience. I'm also a parent, so I have the added bonus of seeing education outside the limited lens of my classroom and in the larger, more realistic view from my dining room table. I know the direct repercussions of too much homework, or inane projects. I see the tears and the triumphs of your day each afternoon when my child unpacks her bag and starts her work.

As a teacher, I know what it means when the year is winding down and I need to finish my curriculum. I know the crunch time before vacation when I need to pile up the homework and make some headway. As a parent, though, I know that prioritizing homework over vacation means schoolwork when I want my kids available for the limited hours we get as a family.

So I've walked that fine line. I know what it means on both sides.

My children have had teachers that inspired them. They have been motivated and given the tools to go on to higher education. They have had teachers who have opened up worlds to them—in books, in science, in math. I'm writing you this letter, though, because you have somehow missed something in your education. Something slipped past the professor who was supposed to teach you classroom methodology. You graduated and you got your degree, and I am sure you have read books upon books about classroom management and differentiated instruction and other educational jargon.

But someone needs to tell you the straight-up truth about teaching. And I have taken it upon myself to point out a few things you need to know for the future. Things I have learned over the years.

You are the attitude and atmosphere in your classroom at all times. But discipline does not need to be angry. Maintaining control in a classroom does not require stern looks and threatening postures. Smiling does not mean that your students will take advantage of you. On the contrary, they will learn the value of a positive attitude. They will trust you. They will feel safe with you. You can balance your authority with love, and you will find that your students will flourish.

They are with you for hours at a time. Make it a point to smile at each one. Sincerely.

You can also be flexible. I have taught seventeen-year-old students who had their computers crash on them or who showed me remnants of projects that had been run over in their driveways. And even though I don't accept late papers, each case is different, and there is a time for compassion and a time to be intractable. You need to know the difference between a student who takes advantage and a student who needs a break. You should have rules. You should have high expectations. But you also need to balance those rules with the realities of life. A wise teacher knows the difference between compassion and weakness and knows when to bend.

You need to also know that one year in the life of a child is enormous. To you, nothing changes—you finish your year, start again, open your books, recite your lessons. But to the students who are in your classroom, that year is a major part of their development. You are the one they will remember when they speak to their own children about school. What story will you be? The one about the worst teacher or the best? Every day, you create that memory for them. Decide who you want to be.

Your students have parents who love them. Who trust you with them for an entire day. You may have students who bother you, with messy hair or unkempt clothes. Maybe a kid with a disorganized backpack. You might have a student with an annoying habit.

That student is someone's entire life.

Always keep that in mind. Because any disparaging comment you make about that child—while chatting in the hallway or walking into the classroom—might be overheard. And in that one second, you have destroyed her, in ways you cannot even fathom. And to a parent, that is unforgivable. It is your job to keep her safe from the mean kids. You can't become one. Even in private. Because you think that the students don't know, but they do.

Dear Teacher, your job is to teach. But in the hours you spend in front of your class you are responsible for so much more than just your curriculum. The way you teach fractions is so much more vital than the content of your lessons. The way you return homework is so much more educational than the red pen marks across the page. The way you carry yourself each day in front of that class will define your success and the success of your students.

Because, dear teacher, your professor no doubt forgot to tell you that happy students learn better than fearful students.

Your class may be lined up in rows, and your students may be marching in lines and raising their hands, but if they are not smiling in your room, then you have failed.

And then you are not a teacher.

First Day

Another school year is about to start. The school supplies are purchased and packed in different-colored backpacks. The uniforms are clean and there are no worn-out knees in the crisp blue slacks. The last few days of summer barbecues and swimming have ended, and now it's time for books and homework, studying and organized sports.

When I was a new teacher, I didn't fully appreciate the impact I had on the students that walked through my door. More importantly, I didn't understand the world each one of them represented to someone else. It wasn't until I was at my first graduation that I had a glimpse into that. Right before the graduates walked down the aisle, baby pictures of each student were displayed on the screens in front of the guests. Seeing those seventeen- and eighteen-year-olds as small children reminded me that I was in charge of someone else's baby. Those kids drove me crazy, and they were aggravating to deal with, but they had parents who loved them. Parents who worked so hard to see them grow up. Parents who knew them when they were young, and cute, and innocent.

My responsibility had been huge, and I don't think I realized it until the year had ended and my students were graduates. But I have since then.

Having children of my own has changed that perspective further. Over the years, as I handed my kids over to their teachers, I silently prayed that the young, just-out-of-college educators would realize what I was giving them. As the teacher smiled sweetly from the door, I wanted to say, "This is my life. Right here. Walking through your door with her backpack and new pencils. It's my world sitting in that seat." I wanted to tell the teacher to protect her. To be a Mama Bear. To keep her away from the mean girls, to encourage her, to help her grow. To be strong.

But there were always twenty other kids in the class, and so many parents dropping off their charges at the same time that my words would never have meant anything. So I always just waved and smiled and high-fived the other parents on the way out. Yay school!

But I silently worried. And I still do.

The first day is a day of trepidation for me. Even after all these years. Because I know that some teachers just don't get it. They are overworked and underpaid and underappreciated, and my kid is just one of the pack. A name on a roster.

I also know it's a reality that my kids will have to get used to eventually. There will be countless first days in their lives—at work, at college, in new cities. Countless places where their uniqueness will not be noticed.

I wonder if I'll ever get used to it. I mean, it's just another first day. Like every year.

But even with some of my kids in high school, I still find myself praying as they walk out the front door, "This is my life. You have my world. Please take care of them."

It's another first day.

Reading Log Lies

Most nights, I go to sleep wondering if I am teaching my son to lie.

It's true. Straight up. Full disclosure.

Maybe it's because he's the fifth child. Or maybe it's just that I'm older. But every night when I tuck him into bed and he casually reminds me he needs to do his reading log—well, something inside me just dies.

Because I would love to read to him. Truly. I would. I would love to hear him read as well. And he does read to me, and I to him. But the nightly twenty-minute assignment and subsequent signing of some document attesting to such reading is driving me to drink unhealthy amounts of alcohol.

It wasn't always like this.

With my first child, I looked forward to filling out that form. I would sign my name each night and list the titles we read. I scorned the class mom who said that she always signed it, regardless of whether her son did the reading.

I would *never* do that, I thought. What poor parenting!

I was the only mom who kept the chart unsigned on the days we did not read. My daughter, distraught, would pick up anything that would count as "reading," just so I would fill out the form before we got in the car.

"Mom! I read the cereal box for five minutes! Please sign my reading log!"

But I didn't. Because I thought I would be teaching her to lie.

Of course, as the only child in her class who had a mom that kept it honest, she was also the only kid who did not get a gold star every single day on the "Super Star Readers!" chart. I thought I was laying the firm moral ground she would need as an adult. I thought I was teaching her values.

Fast forward a few years, and I'm practically leading my seven-year-old down a path of fraud and tax evasion because now I sign that paper nightly without thinking twice. I'm tired, I've been on my feet all day, I finally get him into bed after three cups of water and some apple slices -- and then he pulls out that final ace up his sleeve.

No more, teacher. No more.

I know the teacher means well. She wants to make sure the kids read. And that's important, I know. But the truth? I don't think I'm alone in my reading log lies. I'll bet there are legions of mothers and fathers—no doubt mothers and fathers with more than two children, mind you—who have no compunction about scrawling their names on that dreaded chart without cracking open a Maurice Sendak or a Mary Pope Osborne. I am done with the forced reading time and documentation of my library of picture books. Finished with endless lists of dates and page numbers and "minutes read." I will fill out that paper and hand it in with the full knowledge that I am committing some kind of elementary-school perjury, and I embrace that wholeheartedly.

Because I am sure that a larger group of parents sit with their kids each night and slave through pages of homework. I am part of that group. We watch our kids while they do math problem after math problem. We yell at them from the kitchen while we are fixing dinner, and we lose out on so many family moments because we are overprogrammed and overworked and stressed out.

I simply cannot add reading to the list of stresses.

So my son and I have a tacit understanding. He reads. I sign the reading log. When he doesn't read, I still sign the reading log, because he reads anyway. He has books under his bed. He reads on the weekends. And we read together as well. On days that I come home early. On Saturday afternoons and Friday nights. He picks up the books and reads without looking at the clock to make sure he has finished his required reading.

Technically, then, I guess I'm not really lying. I'm just mixing up the dates.

But I'll be damned before he doesn't get a star on the reading chart in his classroom.

Candy Is a Healthy Choice

We have junk in our house. Real junk. Chocolate. Cookies. Lollipops (even the red ones). There are chips and pretzels. Cupcakes, cookies, and Fruity Pebbles.

We eat pizza during the week.

I don't buy organic food unless it's on sale. I don't know the difference between grass-fed meat and the other ones on the shelf.

We eat whole wheat, but we also have white bread.

I bake using flour and sugar.

Before you call Child Protective Services, you should know the flip side of this pantry from nutritional hell.

My kids choose fruit. They love salads as snacks. They ask for carrots in their lunch and remind me when we need more apples. They get annoyed when the grapes aren't washed and ready on the table. For all the awesome cake and cookies, they want vegetables. Go figure.

Our house is also the house where their friends want to hang out. After all, we have the good food. And while their friends go for the chocolate and the donuts, my kids are eating the strawberries and the cantaloupe.

It's a bizarre little paradox. Here I am, going against what all the good mommies preach, and my kids are eating healthy. They aren't obese. They're active. They're not lethargic.

When I was in high school, I used to go to my friend's house in Manhattan Beach. Her neighbor had a drawer in his kitchen that was filled with candy. Not just any candy, but a Halloween treasure trove. Kit Kats, Hershey bars, Nestlé Crunch—the kind of candy I used to dream about. The kids in the house had full access to that drawer.

I was amazed.

Naturally, whenever I was at my friend's house, we went next door, and the first thing I did was open that drawer. I swear, I think I heard angels singing each time it opened. I couldn't understand why it was filled. Because if I lived there? It would be empty by the morning. No question.

I don't have a "candy drawer" in my house, but my kids have access to the good stuff. Still, they make healthy choices, and I'm not sure why. Yesterday, my seven-year-old looked at the cereal on the shelf—Cheerios, Corn Flakes, Froot Loops, Cookie Crisp, Kix—and reached for the box that he always takes: Kix. My daughter ate strawberries. Even with five kids in the house, we rarely finish a box of sugar cereal.

I have a niece and nephew who are not allowed to drink *juice*. I don't think there is any sugar in their home. Ever. Cake is sweetened with prunes.

That's all fine and good, but give one of those kids a sip of OJ and they are swinging from the rooftops. They come to my house and it's like they're in a crack den, hoarding whatever they can find, licking lollipops on the bathroom floor like addicts.

I have seen this everywhere. Parents of small children who treat corn syrup like poison, who fill a piñata with wheat germ and raisins, who tsk-tsk at the moms with juice boxes. These parents swear that their kids will learn to make healthy choices.

I think the reason my kids choose healthy snacks is that they have the *option* to make those choices. There are no angels that sing when they see a candy bar because it isn't a big deal. Never touching candy creates kids that are obsessed with sugar, that dream of one day having chocolate that doesn't have random seeds in it. Kids that salivate when someone takes out orange juice. Kids that will one day be crushing Smarties and snorting them in lines.

Okay, maybe not that last one. But you never know.

Granted, there are certain things I won't buy. Cakes that have more calories than one is supposed to have in a day. Food with so much fat that it might as well come with a Lipitor prescription. Sticky things, like Fruit Roll-Ups, that stay on teeth and quickly cause cavities. Those things stay on the supermarket shelves.

But I have no problem with chips. Or cookies. In fact, based on my experience, it seems that junk food is the gateway drug to healthy food.

Imagine that.

Everything in moderation, I guess.

Off to Camp

The bags are packed. The duffels have shipped. The stationery and envelopes have been carefully organized and prestamped.

My daughter is leaving for sleep-away camp.

It's her first time going, but it's not my first time sending a kid away for a summer. I know what to do. I've marked her clothing using both iron-on labels and indelible ink in hopes that the clothing will actually return in her bags at the end of the month. I've taught her the nuances of the "laundry bag"—pin your socks, don't throw in anything wet—even though I know she will still return with moldy clothes and virtually no matching pairs of socks. She has shampoo and soap, toothpaste and toothbrushes. ("Take an extra, just in case!") I label a handy-dandy shower caddy for her to keep her things in. She has her summer reading books for school. Her duffel bag is organized and compartmentalized to help her unpack when she gets to her bunk.

Didn't kids once go off with a bundle tied to a stick?

It's kind of a game. Having done this before, I know what is going to happen when she gets to her bunk. I know how my carefully planned and executed packing and preparing for camp will be for naught. I'll see her in pictures on the camp website wearing clothes I don't recognize, and I'll find that jacket she begged me to send to camp on the back of a bunkmate. I'll pore over the pictures and enlarge her teeth to make sure that yes, they have been brushed. At least once. I'll wonder if that spot on her neck is dirt or just the camera lens. And why is her face so red? Didn't she remember the sunscreen?

No matter how much I prepare and send with her, the bottom line is, she is off on her own. I know she won't shower as much as she should. I know the counselors will probably empty half her toothpaste in the sink the night before visiting day so I will believe she brushed often and effectively. I know she won't break the binding on her book, and summer reading will be crammed in during the week before school starts. And I know that half her clothes will be lost, destroyed, or moldy.

Even though I try to pack every comfort of home, summer camp is more than just relocating. I can prepare her all I want, but once she's out there, well, there's no telling what she'll do. And that's okay. Because even though I'm creating this guise of concern for her hygiene and education, I'm actually much more interested in seeing a smile on her face.

Summer camp is time away. It's time away from technology and TV, cell phones and iPads. It's time away from the nagging of Mom and Dad and the fights with siblings. And for some, it's time away from showers and toothbrushing and clean clothes. I've made peace with that. Because camp is really about listening to ghost stories and turning on flashlights with your bunkmates. It's screaming at the bugs and the heat, and creating memories. It is so much more than the organized camp list and duffel.

My kids take turns going to camp. With five kids, sending all of them at once would cost as much as a second mortgage, and my husband and I decided a long time ago that having a house was more important than a few weeks in a bunk. Their experiences have been mixed. My oldest son loved it. My second daughter, not so much. Though, granted, that was the summer of swine flu, and she spent most of her time in the infirmary or home. This summer, it is my youngest daughter's turn.

I hope she has a great time this summer. I hope she writes letters and wishes it would last longer. And I hope she appreciates my efforts to send her away prepared to survive the wilds without me there to help her.

But that last bit is a fantasy. Maybe even the letters part. After sending three other kids off for the summer, I've learned not to expect much in the way of appreciation for my painstakingly neurotic packing and preparing. In fact, they probably would've been happier with less.

But at least I know that she has what she needs. That I have done my job. That she is armed with toothpaste, sunscreen, and bug spray as she goes to live in the wilds of her newly renovated bunk.

Even though, in reality, what she will use at camp could probably fit in a bundle tied to a stick.

And that's all good.

For My Daughter, on Her Eighteenth Birthday

I've written recommendations for hundreds of students and helped them write their essays for college. I've helped them apply for jobs, internships, and summer programs. But ask me to come up with a few words about my own kid, and I'm drawing a blank.

Maybe it's because you are my oldest. You are the child that transformed me into "Mom" and the one that paved the way for your siblings. Your dad and I didn't know what we were doing when they handed you to us. Frankly, I couldn't believe they let me take you out of the hospital without even looking up my background or checking my fingerprints. But there I was, holding this miracle who didn't come with any instruction manual, save the unspoken understanding that if you cried, I would find out why.

And so, as we hurtled through the years, we learned. You were the constantly changing blueprint that we based our later decisions on. You taught us about what was normal, and what wasn't. When your siblings came around, we based their stages and milestones on the benchmarks you

51

set. It was our only experience, and we learned through you. You received the brunt of our early parenting mistakes and watched us mellow out as the others grew.

You are, I guess, a typical first child. Hardworking, motivated, focused. We can't take any responsibility for that, though. It was hardwired into you since birth. Maybe you knew how unsure we were, and so you unconsciously took over. I never had to remind you to do your homework. Never had to worry about lost papers. Never had to tell you to clean your room. You were on top of everything. Even when you became a teenager, I never had to worry about curfews or strict rules. You went to bed on time and never understood how people could function the next day without enough hours of sleep. You were also rarely content to just sit around. Even now, your days are planned, your activities organized, and your goals firmly in sight.

I look at you with awe sometimes. Not believing that you were the baby they put into my arms so long ago. Not equating this self-assured young woman with the girl who loved watching *Teletubbies* and *Little Bear* and waited for Peter Pan to fly through her window. I was warned that the years would fly by, and now, eighteen years later, I finally understand. I'm watching you apply for college, and that tired metaphor about spreading your wings and flying actually makes sense. You're getting ready to leap out into the world, and I am both terrified and proud.

In short, you amaze me. Perhaps it's because you are my daughter and my oldest. Because every step you take is always new. Because you astound me with your maturity and your tenacity. But really, it's because you are such a better person at eighteen than I was at that age, and I know that if I were in your class, I would want to be your friend.

But I know, I'm your mom. What else would I say, right?

I don't have words of wisdom for you on this, your eighteenth birthday. No Polonius speeches about being a borrower or a lender. You have been a proven product: in your decisions, your choices, and your drive. The only advice that suits you now is just to continue on. Continue to amaze me. Continue to blaze a path. Continue to make your life epic.

You are so much more than I can put on paper because you are constantly doing more than I ever expected.

And you are everything to me.

Happy birthday.

"It's a Ceremony!"

It's the season of graduations, and my newsfeed is filled with caps and gowns and diplomas. This year, I had two kids doing the "Pomp and Circumstance" walk. One was graduating from high school and the other finishing middle school. They were beautiful ceremonies, filled with speeches and video montages and weeping parents bursting with pride.

I wasn't alone, of course. And my kids' graduations weren't unique. In the week that they graduated from their respective schools, I saw posts from kindergarten graduations, pre-K graduations, fifth-grade graduations, and, God help us all, third-grade graduations. There were tons of "moving-up" ceremonies, kids crossing the hallway into new classrooms in proceedings replete with gowns (but no hats) and heartfelt speeches.

It reminded me of that scene from *The Incredibles* when Mr. Incredible, exasperated by his son's "graduation" from fourth grade to fifth, yells "It's psychotic!"

And in truth, he has a point.

A graduation marks a milestone. Finishing high school and starting college. Out of middle school and into high school. But all the mini-graduations that have silently insinuated themselves into schools across the country have made these larger moments seem less significant. Worse, by celebrating every nuanced moment in education, kids learn that they should always be celebrated, even when it might not be warranted.

I'm not saying it isn't cute. Watching four-year-olds in caps and gowns certainly provides great Instagram moments. But as a larger issue—one that Mr. Incredible bemoaned in that same scene—are we simply looking for "new ways to celebrate mediocrity?"

Because let's be real. Discussing a four-year-old's accomplishments as he gets a diploma borders on ridiculousness. Finishing fourth grade doesn't require a ceremony. At most, maybe some ice cream and balloons and a "Good Luck Next Year!" banner.

I get eighth grade. I get twelfth grade. I can even get kindergarten. (Though graduating pre-K disturbs me on a grammatical level. How can you graduate anything that is "pre"? That prefix alone implies another step! Jeez!) But all these end-of-the-year ceremonies have gotten out of hand.

It also adds undue stress. I remember my big transition to middle school years ago. It consisted of moving across the hall, with a quick memo reminding us that we would switch classes throughout the day. That was it. One year I was in fifth. The next year I was in sixth and I needed a Trapper Keeper.

Now, there's a "graduation" from fifth grade, a constant reminder that even though you might be just across the hall, you are in a whole new world! And this is *much* harder! And you might be stressed!

Seriously?

I mean, it's possible you'll be nervous. Just as any new year presents new things to be nervous about. New teachers.

New friends. New lockers. It's called growing up. It's called reaching for a goal. It's called climbing the educational ladder. There are milestones to that journey, and they don't always come every year or every semester.

My kids have had graduations for years. I have all the school pictures and the family shots from pre-K and on, dutifully posted with "I'm so proud of my baby!" captions. But this last one—watching my daughter finish high school—was the only time I felt that it was truly a graduation. A valediction. That she was really going off into the world. That she had accomplished something, not over four years, but over twelve.

I'm definitely coming from a jaded perspective. I was much more excited when my oldest "graduated" kindergarten. Much less so when my youngest walked across the pre-K stage to get his diploma in paper-cutting, shape-making, and block center. Watching my kids go through school allowed me to see past the Instagram pics and focus on what is really important in their education, in their lives, and in their milestones.

My mother used to tell me that your perspective on child-rearing can't extend beyond your oldest child. Experience teaches us so much more than the textbooks and articles. In some ways, then, my daughter's graduation from high school is also my own graduation into a new stage of parenting.

So, with apologies to all the newly minted pre-K kids, all the proud parents of the third-grade commencements, and all the fifth graders moving up, this new frontier I have been launched into makes me wonder if all those years of graduations really were nothing more than photo ops. Sort of a metaphorical pat on the back for simply going to school. Cute and sweet, though over time perhaps wearisome and boring.

This year, I'm celebrating two actual graduations (not including my own).

And damn, I am proud.

Nature of the Beast

I lost my eighteen-month-old daughter at Disney World.

No, this isn't some urban legend like you read about. She wasn't kidnapped, drugged, and discovered at the gate with a stranger and newly dyed hair.

She wandered off, and we didn't see.

We were at Disney with my brother and his family and my good friend and her family. All in all, we were a group of thirteen. I rented a stroller, and since it had a convenient canopy, everyone in the party promptly tossed their backpacks and jackets on top of it.

No big deal. I was used to it. It was one of the perks of having a stroller in the park.

We were walking from Splash Mountain to Pirates of the Caribbean, and we stopped for a few moments to watch a passing marching band. In those few seconds—about ten, to be specific—my eighteen-month-old daughter escaped the seatbelt and walked out of the stroller. With everyone's bags on top of the stroller, I didn't even feel the weight differential when she stepped out. And so, we continued on.

At Pirates of the Caribbean, I turned the stroller around and was horrified to find it empty.

Keep in mind, there were thirteen of us. No one saw her get up and run off. No one saw her get out of the stroller. No one realized she was missing until we arrived in Adventureland.

Of course, this has a happy ending. My brother ran back to Splash Mountain, I grabbed a Disney employee, and within minutes she was found, safely wandering through some kiosk, happily oblivious.

It's a story we retell, laughing and joking about how ridiculous it was. I've used the story to caution others who rent strollers ("Don't pile everything on top!"). And my daughter has heard it over and over again. Especially whenever we go to Disney.

Of course, she didn't fall into a gorilla compound.

I've been thinking of when the internet blasted the mother of the young boy who fell into that compound, accusing her of neglect and demanding prosecution and the removal of her other children. Parents posted Facebook updates announcing that they *never* let their children out of their sight. *Never* would let that happen to them.

I was stunned.

Ironically, at the same time the internet was decrying the mother of this poor boy, there were other articles in my newsfeed criticizing helicopter parents, the ones who never let their kids play in dirt ("Germs!"), or walk down the block ("Stranger Danger!"), or lose at a game ("Self-Esteem!").

You can't have it both ways, people.

The ER is filled with "neglectful" parents whose children need stitches after falling on the playground, or who swallowed too much bubblegum-flavored Motrin after suddenly discovering they could open it. And whether it was preventable or not, there is always an element of guilt that plays out.

Neglectful parenting? Not if you've actually been a parent for more than fifteen minutes. Good parents know that childhood is fraught with the unexpected bolt from the stroller, the quick grab of the medicine, the split second of missed footing on the slide. Good parents know these things happen, and usually they become the stuff of family legends, retold and embellished at gatherings and bar mitzvahs.

Rarely do the stories involve the media and a dead gorilla.

As tragic as the story is, placing the blame squarely on the mother puts every other parent who has ever had to tend to skinned knees in that "neglectful parent" category as well. And while it's true that my kid never climbed over the fence in the zoo, I can see how something like that can happen in the split second it takes for a four-year-old to bolt.

It's the nature of the beast.

Auschwitz Today

When my oldest daughter studied abroad during her first year of college, she had the opportunity to visit Poland. Prior to going, she spent some time learning about the Jewish history of the areas she would visit, the life that was there both before and during World War II. She even emailed me before she left, asking for some family history so she could relate to the cities and graveyards she was going to see.

I never went to Poland, but I have seen pictures of high-school students on the *March of the Living* or on *Heritage Seminars,* programs that take Jewish kids from across the globe to Poland to learn firsthand about the history that shaped their culture. The pictures all look the same. Kids in front of Auschwitz. Kids at Majdanek. There is always the shot of a student draped in an Israeli flag, their back to the camera, walking with friends along the train tracks leading to Auschwitz.

"You need to take that picture," I told my daughter, and she immediately knew which one I was talking about.

"No, Mom. I'm not."

"Yes! You have to!"

"Everyone takes that picture!"

"I know! You have to! At least now I'll know the person behind the flag!"

But she really didn't want to. Too clichéd. Too overdone. But then, a few days into her trip, she sent me the picture I wanted. There she was, draped in an Israeli flag, walking along the train tracks to Auschwitz. It was the overdone, overexposed shot.

And it left me breathless.

Because even though I had seen that setup so many times, I wasn't prepared for the emotional punch of seeing my own kid in that place. Walking on train tracks that led millions to their deaths. Walking through rooms that might have housed the last moments of my ancestors.

And there she was, nineteen years old, dressed in a red coat and wrapped in an Israeli flag, marching through those gates. Free, vibrant, alive.

The clichéd picture that we had joked about became a powerful symbol for me. A visual of family tradition, a representation of all that was lost in the Holocaust, an image of strength and endurance. I had seen that picture so many times, but knowing it was her, my daughter, put an entirely new spin on it.

I imagined people walking beside her, silently watching this strong Jewish woman. She is ready to take on the world, sure and confident. It reminded me of what was lost. Of the millions who were just like her so many years ago, walking through those gates with no option of leaving. It was a picture that cried out the heavy responsibility she has as a member of the Jewish people, as a moral, upright person in the world, and as my daughter, a link in our family chain.

I called her up soon after I saw the picture. I told her how awesome it was.

"Yeah. Great. Just like everyone else's."

And we laughed and spoke about the food and how tired she was.

When I hung up, I said a silent prayer that she would be kept safe and happy.

And I swear I heard distant voices joining in.

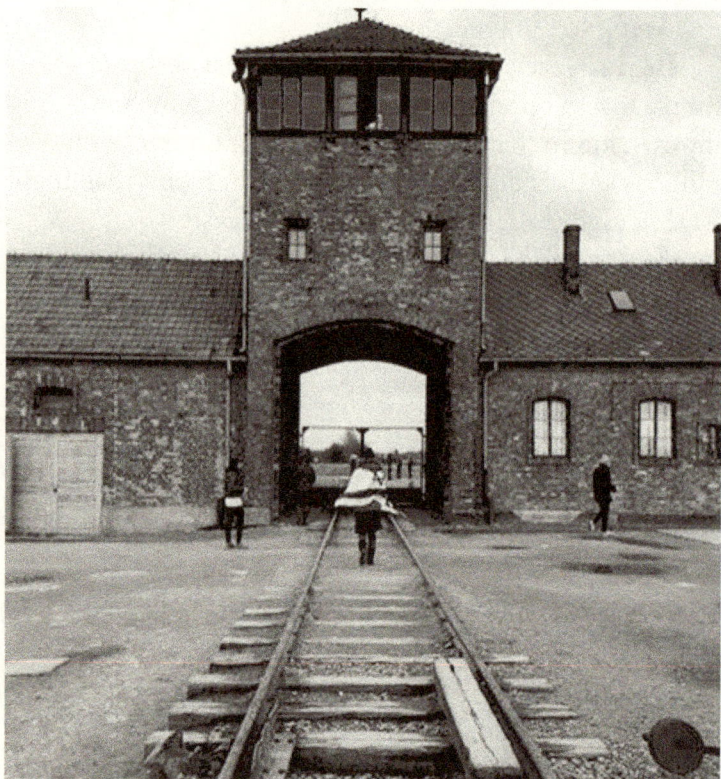

It's the Space Station! Again. And Again

The International Space Station passed over my house at six thirty in the morning. It didn't cause a sonic boom, or disrupt cable or cell phone service. It was just a tiny speck, looking as unremarkable as all the other stars in the early morning sky. But this star moved.

I dragged my kids out of bed to see.

"Look how cool!"

"It's the Space Station!"

"Everybody wave!"

I had also alerted my neighbors, who stood on the street in their pajamas, to watch this incredible cosmic event. I filmed it. Shared it on social media. It was so cool.

But then I discovered it really wasn't as cool as I had thought.

I found the ISS viewing times through a friend of mine who signs up for NASA alerts. You can do this too, by the way, if you register at the Spot the Station website. You enter your location, and NASA will send you an alert indicating where you can catch a glimpse of the Space Station.

So I signed up.

Since last week, when I watched the Space Station pass overhead amid the fanfare and excitement on my little street, I have since received three notifications of viewing opportunities from my front lawn. Space Station sightings, it seems, are rather common. In fact, according to my friend at work who loves science, they are a dime a dozen.

I was a bit crestfallen.

I mean, there I was, dragging my kids out of their beds to show them something they can see any old time? And c'mon, it was just a moving star. Not that exciting anyway. What was I thinking? Especially when I found out how often one can witness this scintillating event.

NASA is making a huge mistake with this Spot the Station website. They should lie. Seriously. They should say that witnessing this is a "once in a very long time" opportunity. Like an eclipse. Because with space shuttle launches a thing of the past, what do we still have that can put a sense of wonder in a kid's mind? Or an adult's, for that matter? I watched the International Space Station pass by and felt like I was witnessing something amazing. I was a part of some global project! Me, on my little street, with my neighbors and my kids, just looking up in awe at a tiny dot that represented how far we have come as a society.

My disappointment after receiving the next two alerts reminded me of how easily jaded I have become.

So here's what I hope. I hope NASA lies. I hope they stop sending out so many alerts and just keep some of that information secret. Let us plebeians here on the ground get a glimpse of a piece of magic that isn't tainted by overexposure.

Because I still want to be excited about space stations.

Summer Reading

It seems that teachers have forgotten what summer vacation means. I have only recently noticed the subtle switch from the summer break of yesteryear to the summer prep period that it has become today. More and more schools are sending their students off in June, not with a sense of completion and relief after a hard year's work, but with enough assignments to swiftly squash any dreams of lazy summer days on the hammock. Students go to camp with textbooks to annotate, novels to write about, and essays to analyze. They bring their books to their places of work and spend significant time, not outside in the sun, but in front of computer screens and notebooks.

At least, that is what the teachers hope.

Truth is, in this age of instant gratification and high-tech wizardry, most students will not tackle those assignments with the vigor teachers hope for. Instead, books are SparkNoted, answer keys are purchased online, and essays are downloaded. Or written by AI.

I don't particularly blame them. A quick look at the average summer assignments in any given school reads like a minicourse curriculum. Read five books for one class and write three essays. Buy two science textbooks and annotate six chapters. Be prepared for a quiz the first day of class on the first three chapters in the math text. My personal favorite was an assignment out of a school in Iowa that demanded a comprehensive project mapping the history of philosophy since the Bible. Based, of course, on the summer reading.

Have teachers lost their minds?

If my principal asked me to read a few educational journal articles over the summer, I would agree that it's a good idea to stay updated and informed. If he asked me to read the articles, answer a set of fifty questions, and be prepared for a quiz that would affect my midyear review, I'd show him a particular body part he could kiss.

Summer vacation was always a chance to unwind, relax, and recharge for another year. It was a time to get some real-world experiences as well—travel, work, fun. There were always summer assignments, but they were usually limited to "Choose a book from the following list and write a summary." The objective was simple: teachers just wanted students to keep their minds going. They wanted them to read a good book or two. Now, the schoolwork kids are doing over the summer seems to only serve the teacher, who can claim demanding classes and high expectations. Or the work serves overbearing parents who need to show off the difficult work their child is capable of. Maybe it makes them feel that the kid has a head start into the college world.

It's hard to say that it benefits the student. A true benefit would be to let them enjoy their summer, practice what they learned in the real world, and develop a sense of what they truly want to do with their lives. Don't set them up for failure on the first day of school by giving them work over the summer that assumes they are doing nothing important.

Fun is important. Leisure is important. Lying on a hammock is important.

Annotating *Frankenstein*, which one school assigned to their tenth grade, is not. That's an assignment that should be handled in school, with a teacher who can guide the students. Give the students a book that is current, that will engage them and inspire them to read more. Give them books that don't require teaching but instead just generate the "you must read this!" response. The kind of texts that kids *want* to discuss, not the ones they are *required* to discuss.

That is a summer assignment that will create lifelong readers and thinkers.

My ten-year-old daughter has to read three books and write three book reports over the next four weeks. She recently asked if she could just google the books and write the summaries from there.

How quickly they learn. I just wish the teachers would.

In J. J. Abrams We Trust

It took me a week after *Star Wars: The Force Awakens* blew up box office records to brave Twitter and Facebook and Instagram again, no longer worried about spoilers. I had seen the film twice in that time. The first time was a serious "Oh my God I'm watching Star Wars again" event. The second time around, I was a bit more critical, but I still had that excitement. Still had that new movie rush.

Going to the movie really was like going back to that first time I saw *Star Wars*. It was a feeling I wanted my kids to experience as well. After all, this movie represented something larger. It was like being part of a historic moment. Selling that idea, though, proved to be a bit of a challenge.

I was clear from the start: we were going to see the movie as a family.

I bought everyone T-shirts.

We hummed the theme song in carpool. We played the trailer on repeat. For the most part, the kids all joined in on the excitement and anticipation.

Everyone except for my thirteen-year-old daughter.

Granted, thirteen-year-olds are not the easiest to convince when it comes to joining in on family events, but this one was particularly contrary. She hadn't watched the older films when I'd insisted everyone else watch them. She hates science fiction.

And she flat out refused to see the movie.

I insisted.

Thus began the great Star Wars Battle of 2015. The more she put up a fight, the more I dug my heels in.

I tried being rational: "This is part of your education."

I tried pulling rank: "You have no choice here. We are seeing it as a family."

I tried guilt: "Do you know how important this is to your mom? Don't you care about that?"

It didn't help that her siblings and my husband started taking sides. Bets were placed to see who would give in. Would I force her to join us, angry and muttering the whole time? Would she relent? Realize it was a lost cause?

My husband was on her side and pointed out the obvious. "She is going to hate it," he said. "She is going to hate it, and then she will never let you forget it. Why are you forcing her? And why do you even want her to come if she will be so miserable?"

A part of me knew he was right. In the great battles of parents vs. teenagers, this one was definitely not worth it. But I was too entrenched in the fight. Too deep in my insistence. Backing off would be giving in, and that wasn't going to happen.

Our tickets were for Saturday night. By Saturday afternoon, she had started to make peace with it.

"Fine," she said. "I'll go. But I won't wear the stupid shirt."

But I saw this as a break in the wall. The caving of her defenses. I was winning this.

"You're going and you're wearing the shirt."

My husband rolled his eyes as my daughter and I went at it again.

"Why do I have to wear the shirt?? I'm going!"

I didn't give in. Again, in retrospect, it was silly of me. But at that point, I was going all the way.

On Saturday night, we were getting ready to leave. She came out of her room wearing the Star Wars shirt.

"I'll wear the shirt and go to the movie. But I am *not* going to be in any of the pictures."

We left for the theater, and that's when I started getting nervous. Because what if she hated it? What if it was terrible? For a moment, I doubted myself. It was only fleeting, though.

She would love it. I was sure. And it had nothing to do with Star Wars or science fiction either. I knew she wouldn't hate it because it was a J. J. Abrams film. And as the lights went down, I silently prayed that he would deliver.

The rest, of course, is obvious.

She loved the movie. Thanked me for taking her. Said it was really good. She asked questions and I filled her in. She loved Rey. Loved Han. Loved the effects. (Though she thought the transitions between scenes were terrible. I explained that they were "retro." She still felt they could have done better.)

In the Great Star Wars Battle of 2015, I clearly won. But there was no gloating on my part. No nasty, annoying, mom-like expressions of "I told you so." My victory played out in a much more subtle way.

I took my family to see *Star Wars*. We shared a moment in history. We swapped theories. We argued and critiqued.

And my thirteen-year-old daughter proudly took pictures with her geek mom.

And let me post it on Instagram.

Matzah and Wine and Switching the Living Room with the Dining Room

When I was young, Passover meant the glasses with the disappearing pattern. They were small with a red and blue design, and they were filled at the seder, the long, drawn-out evening meal where we would retell the story of the exodus from Egypt. The blue would get lost in front of the deep purple grape juice, the red just barely perceptible beside it. We only had a few of them, but I loved choosing those cups for myself. For me, those glasses meant it was Passover.

Passover comes with its own set of strict rules. It isn't just about eating unleavened bread, or *chametz*. All dishes and ingredients and anything that could have come into contact with bread during the year must be put away for the eight days of the holiday. So there were other items as well. Objects that we used once a year, unboxed in our kitchen late at night or early in the morning, appearing on newly cleaned shelves for the week of the holiday. Special bowls that belonged to my grandmothers. A funny-shaped spoon that I loved to use to make chocolate milk. A hand mixer, a nut grater, an apple chopper that seemed to come

71

from the shtetl. They were treasures rediscovered year after year, but the feelings surrounding them never got old. The anticipation of seeing them never waned.

Passover was a magical time when I was a child. I would go to sleep late after we finished the formal search for the *chametz*, a process of symbolically ensuring there was no unleavened bread in the home, and when I awoke the next day, our kitchen would be transformed into a tinfoil-covered wonderland. My mother would stand at the stove with a pot that could easily bathe an average-sized child, cutting vegetables for a chicken soup. I have clear memories of my older sister peering out of the kitchen cabinets. She would line them with paper for the new dishes that waited in the boxes to be used for that one week of the year, and I remember complaining that it was unfair that I never got to climb into the cabinets like she did.

Most Passover traditions are universal. Everyone leans at the table, asks the four questions, and opens the door for Elijah, the prophet who supposedly shows up at everyone's meal on Passover. The seder itself is a sensory experience—the tear-inducing smell of the bitter herbs, the crisp feel of the matzah, the careful glancing (but no pointing!) toward the shank bone, the unique songs, and of course, the taste of everything, from the saltwater tears to the four cups of wine. But some other traditions are unique from family to family. They are the distinct symbols that take one back to Passovers past—the colored cups for me, the special tablecloth for someone else—the symbols that say, "This is Passover." Moreso than the wine and the matzah.

When I first started having my own seders in my home, my collection of unique Passover traditions grew slowly. One of them, though, was completely unintentional. Our seders required adding an extension to our dining room table. So in the interest of comfort, we swapped our dining room with our living room, moving the couches into a smaller area and eating our meals in the larger living room space. It was a practical decision to make our guests (and our meal) more comfortable, and we did it every year.

However, our current house has a much larger dining room. As the preparations for Passover that first year in our new home were winding down, my daughter asked me when we would be transferring the dining room to the living room. I told her we didn't need to; there was enough space in the new house. She looked at me with a look of absolute horror, as if I had suggested we forgo the matzah and just eat bread.

And with that, I realized that the room transformation was her blue-and-red glass. It was what "made" it Passover. The feelings, the vibe, the clear demarcation that Passover had come to the home was the moment that our dining room magically appeared in the living room.

Traditions create the ambience of Passover. They are like fairy dust, sprinkling magic into the holiday in a way that the tinfoil coverings and unique glasses did for me as a child. Religious observances are difficult. It is not easy to sell a toddler on matzah pizza when they are crying for a bagel. It is not easy to stay awake at a seder, to cook ridiculous amounts of food for so many people for so many meals. But the memories of Passover are sweet because of the feelings we create around those observances. The memories we unpack each year, the feelings the objects evoke, and the sense of family and tradition they create tell stories in a much more powerful way than the Haggadah. It's why I have special dishes for Passover. It's why I make once-a-year recipes. It's why we sing unique family tunes at the seder.

And it's why, even though we don't have to, we always swap our living room with our dining room.

It Doesn't Get Any Easier

My second-oldest child left home last week, hopping on a plane to spend a gap year in Israel before she starts college. The year before, I sent my oldest daughter off on pretty much the same trip, so you'd think I would know what I was doing. I followed the same pattern and the same schedule. Shopping. Trips to Target. Electronics stores. Unlocking cell phones and organizing passports and credit cards. We went through the same preflight panic when we realized one of the bags was too heavy and one might not fit the standard carry-on criteria.

And we said our goodbyes.

You'd think that having done this before, I would find it easier, much like watching my children graduate from kindergarten. The first time was beautiful and sentimental. The fifth time, we arrived late and didn't stick around for the cake at the after-party. But instead, leaving my daughter at the airport was heart wrenching. Watching her go off, just like her sister did a year before, was emotional and difficult.

I wasn't sure why. In fact, when friends approached me the next day, they all said the same thing. "Oh, this is probably nothing for you. You're used to this."

It couldn't be further from the truth.

I went bungee jumping when I was eighteen, and I remember leaping headfirst off the platform, 150 feet in the air. I didn't see much of the ground rushing up to meet me because before I knew it, I was springing back toward the platform, terrified that I was going to hit it. And then I went down again. That second time, falling back toward the water, was infinitely more terrifying. I had already done the hard part—I had focused myself, taken a breath, and dived into nothingness. But falling back down after that first jump, when I was jolted uncontrollably back upward after coming within inches of the water, I knew what was coming. I knew what I was falling into. And I knew there was no way to stop and catch my breath.

I think that's why the second time is always harder.

I am now intimately aware of what my daughter getting on that plane means for my family. I know that from this point on, when she comes home, she is only here as a visitor. I know that the family dynamic will shift once again, more dramatically this time with two kids away—one in Israel and one in college. While I knew all these things when my oldest first took off, it hit me slowly, as the year unfolded. When I sat in her room and looked at her posters. When we spoke on WhatsApp. When we FaceTimed and counted the days to her return, only to pack her up and send her off again.

This time, it isn't theoretical. I have no illusions about what it means when my second daughter boards that plane. I'm on that bungee cord hurtling out of control, knowing what's coming and thinking with all my heart, please slow down. So even though I've been at this gate before, the tears come easier this time around, the pain stabs a bit sharper, and the moment becomes significantly more bitter than sweet.

I know when it is my other children's turns, it won't be any easier. Those airport moments will always be hard, no matter how many times I escort a child to the gate, kiss them on the cheek, and wave goodbye.

It doesn't get any easier. That's for sure.

But watching them become independent? Grow? Flourish? That couldn't get any better.

PATIENT

It started with a lump, but the lump turned out to be no big deal. It was 2014. I had two kids in High School, two kids in Middle School, and one in elementary.

I remember telling my friend that it added insult to injury when the sonographer told me that the reason for my concern was "just fat."

"Couldn't they come up with a different name? A scientific name?"

But while looking at that lump—that fat—she found something else. Two tiny little "disturbances in the force." A biopsy revealed some atypical cells. Not cancer. Just some cells that could be a precursor to cancer later on. No big deal.

"Meet with a surgeon to review your options," the doctor said. "You should probably have those two spots removed. Simple outpatient procedure."

No big deal.

The surgeon agreed that I should have the procedure. Two tiny little spots. Remove them, and then just keep following up. But she recommended I get an MRI as well.

"Let's just get the whole picture," she said. "No big deal."

The MRI revealed a much larger, six-inch "disturbance in the force" that a mammogram and ultrasound did not pick up. They did another two biopsies of the area and came back with more atypical cells.

"But," the surgeon said, "even though we didn't find cancer cells, we don't know. It's a huge area. You need to remove it."

And the only way to remove a six-inch area from a breast is to remove the entire breast. They recommended removing both.

No big deal.

I wasn't buying it. If they didn't find cancer, then there was no way I was going to do this major surgery. I had seen the movies. I knew how you were supposed to get cancer. Someone sits you in a room, sighs deeply, and says, "Girl, you have cancer." But this? I'm going to get my breasts removed on the *possibility* of there being cancer? No.

I went to five different doctors from different cities and states, looking for someone to tell me not to do the surgery. It didn't make sense to me. But no one agreed. They all said the same thing: "Do the surgery. In the long run, it's your safest bet."

I went to that surgery kicking and screaming. But I did it anyway, thinking I was making a terrible error.

Three days later, the surgeon called me to let me know that they found three invasive tumors in my breast. Suddenly, I needed an oncologist. Suddenly, I was having conversations about treatment options. Suddenly, I was a cancer patient.

And nothing was ever the same after that.

No big deal.

The Beach at Night

I went to the beach at night.

There was something poetic about the whole thing. It played out in my head like a scene from a movie. Close-up of the protagonist, wind in her hair, staring out into the vast, deep ocean. Stars overhead, full moon, the waves crashing onto the sand. Slow, melodramatic piano solo in the background.

In the movie version, of course, whatever concern prompted the main character to ponder the sea is soon solved. The answers roll onto shore as easily as the waves.

I left the chaos of bedtime and homework and walked on the sand, waiting for something. A sign. An epiphany. Maybe a helpful stranger who had all the answers. A kindly vagrant, even. A wise old man.

But while I waited for every movie trope I could think of, none of them made their appearance on the beach that night. It was just me and the sand, the sea, the stars, and the unanswered questions lingering in the air.

I sat down and closed my eyes, listening intently to the ocean. Searching for some secret answer that might wash up. Listening to whatever secrets danced on the wind.

I focused. Meditated a bit. Tried to find something from inside myself. Reached back into my mind and pulled at the straws that lay scattered there.

The ocean soothed my soul. With my eyes closed, I could pretend whatever I wanted. Be whoever I wanted. Imagine myself somewhere else. Just for a moment, that is.

There were decisions to make. Plans to follow. So many dreams and hopes. And there on the beach, under the stars, I willed them into existence. I embraced the sky, the stars, the surf, and begged for wings. I took flight, right then and there. I soared effortlessly, and I landed in a cradle of unseen comfort that washed over me in moon rays and echoes.

But then, I opened my eyes.

My mind was far from clear. It was filled with all the stresses of the day. Of the month. Of a year interrupted. They were still there as I sat in the sand, alone, at night, on the beach. My phone lit up with concerned texts. "Where did you go? Are you okay?"

I had only been there a few minutes. After all, the beach in my movie was very different from reality. In the real world, the vagrants aren't too friendly. The wandering old men aren't disguised wizards. The sea is quicker to wash up discarded plastic than clarity and peace.

Serenity is easy to find with your eyes shut tight, but eventually, you have to open them , deal, and forge on. Without imaginary wings or phantom guides or moonlit pathways.

I went to the beach at night, and I left the same way I arrived.

Just reality. Alone on the beach.

Not exactly the movie version I'd gone looking for, but maybe what I found was precisely the answer I needed.

Fade to black.

Redefining "Fine"

Each time I sit down to write, I try to avoid the elephant sitting next to me that demands a forum.

It's been tough to ignore. And trust me, I am well schooled in the art of denial. I'm practically the poster child for it.

It might be why, when I found a lump in my breast, I assumed it was nothing. And actually, that was true. But the rest of what was found there, after the ultrasounds and the MRIs and the biopsies, turned out to be more than nothing. Each day changed the situation. It went from "This is nothing" to "This might be something" to "You'll be fine, we caught it early."

I quickly became educated in the sliding scale that is "fine" and how that scale changes when you're sitting in an oncologist's office. "Fine" used to mean Neosporin and a Band-Aid. Now, it means surgery, maybe some radiation, but I'll live. It's like suddenly getting thrust into the alternate 1985 in *Back to the Future*. Only there is no time machine to fix this, no Doc Brown to find 1.21 gigawatts of power.

Thank you for that heaping serving of perspective with my morning coffee.

It could be worse. I know that. It's what I tell the people who look at me with weepy eyes and want to hug me. I don't need any of that. After all, I'm FINE. Or the well-meaning, encouraging friends who tell me I can fight this when they don't realize that at this point, it's a passive fight. It's a civil war within myself, and I'm letting the armies fall back and hoping they don't leave any cellular spies behind. It's a fight that plays out in operating rooms and MRI machines and consists of me lying prone while getting stabbed multiple times. Always followed by, "You're fine."

I've spoken to many people, friends of friends, who have gone down this same path and have echoed that sentiment. And then I hear about the others. The ones who aren't "fine." The ones whose prognoses include words like "hospice" and "palliative" and "terminal," nowhere near my own horrible new version of "fine." Those stories slap me in the face, shove me against a wall, and yell, "How dare you complain!" in response to my laughably mild prognosis.

I've sat with my friends and done the math and realized that I am the one in eight from the statistic that I keep hearing. I tell them that we should keep getting together in groups of eight so that they can beat the odds in some kind of twisted *Final Destination* fate game. Hang out with me, and statistically, you will all be better than fine. You will be the seven out of eight.

I am lucky. It has taken some time to wrap my head around that idea, but it's true. I dodged a bullet. This could have been much worse. I might have a difficult year ahead of me, but I will eventually get back to the 1985 I know. And while I don't have plans to turn all my writing into thoughts of cancer and treatments, I know it might dominate some of my reflections as I am launched on this journey.

But I have nothing to mourn. Nothing to cry over. I will

have years and years after this blip on the screen. Years of bringing "fine" back into perspective.

And in the grand scheme of things, that's fine by me.

Waiting Games

In the movies, when someone finds out they have cancer, it happens quickly. Someone is sitting in a doctor's office. Everyone is solemn. The doctor looks at the chart, sighs heavily, and says something poignant like, "Well, it's cancer." Or, "It's malignant." Or, "I'm so sorry."

In reality, there's a lot more waiting involved. And it's the waiting that is the hardest part.

For three months, I've been waiting. Waiting for doctor appointments. Waiting for biopsy results. Waiting for news, good or bad. It's a novel concept in this age of instant gratification. It's intolerable. Foreign. A form of torture that Dante seriously missed, because this waiting placed me squarely in one of the forgotten lower circles of hell.

In oncology offices, surgical suites, and hospital rooms, the waiting exploded with unanswered questions that I couldn't turn off. The intellectual side of my brain reminded me that most of the time, these things work out well. That 85 percent of all biopsies are benign. That everything is fine. But the emotional, irrational part of my brain reminded me that this could be it. The news could be bad. My life was going to change dramatically.

There was no choice but to wait, and that battle played out each day like some kind of psychological smackdown.

"It's nothing!" vs. "It's the end."

"I'm fine." vs. "I'm dying."

No one ever wins, though. Some days it's doom and gloom. Some days it's rainbows and lollipops. But the worst-case scenario always seems to score more points by the end of the day because maybe we are hardwired that way. We assume the worst in a self-preservation effort. Doing so gives us a false sense of preparedness for whatever will come.

Waiting threw me into a black hole of uncertainty. I was Sandra Bullock in *Gravity*, spiraling, and nothing could set me back on course. So I did things that gave me some sense of control. I searched YouTube for videos entitled "Journey of a Biopsy Slide" or "What Happens While You're Waiting?" I called my doctor and pissed off the receptionist with my daily "are those results in yet?" question. I stayed up all night, staring at the ceiling. I obsessively refreshed MyChart.

None of it did anything to stop the constant psychodrama going through my head. I thought I was losing my mind.

Apparently, I wasn't alone. If you want to know how bad waiting can get, someone with stage IV cancer once told me that *waiting* for her results was worse than *finding out* the results.

I found that hard to believe, but I suppose there is a sense of control that comes with a diagnosis. There's a plan. A protocol. The black hole ends, and this time you're in a wormhole, traveling on toward some other course. Even though the destination might be grim, it's better than flying blind.

Right now, I'm flying blind again. I know that I have cancer and I'm waiting on a plan for the rest of the year. But unlike the last few times when I just wanted an answer, I'm not eager to get this news. I'm accepting the uncertainty, embracing the waiting like an old friend. After all, I've been here a few times already.

True, I looked up all the worst-case scenarios. I researched all the drugs. All the side effects. I'm still waiting for the call from the doctor, but I haven't harassed his receptionist yet.

Because at least now I'm not hurtling aimlessly through the black hole of the waiting room in hell. Now, regardless of what they say, I know where this leads to, and I'm aiming straight for it.

And as long as I know the trajectory, the waiting just ain't so bad.

It leads toward life.

On the Shoulders of Wishes

Pain, and the management of it, is consuming most of my time since my surgery. It's a vicious cycle. I wake up in some sort of primeval agony and wait for the two pills that promise relief.

That's the easy pain. It's tangible. It "demands to be felt," like John Green says. And so with every twinge, every pull, every throb, I knock back two pills, and soon I'm enveloped in a warm sea of relief. It clouds my head, denies me lucidity, and man, it is sweet. It lets me walk from my bed to a chair and feel somewhat fulfilled with that little trek. It lets me speak without getting winded. These are magic pills I would easily sell the family cow for, just like in a fairy tale, and I look at the clock to make sure I don't miss the deadline when they start wearing off so I can take two more.

Because the pain in between is worse. That's the moment when my head clears a bit, but my physical ailments are still at bay. It's the time when I can think about the things I don't want to think about. It's the Philip Seymour Hoffman moments where I can imagine taking a few pills too many and transporting myself somewhere else. It's the "Woe-is-me" moment. The moment of "Why?" and "How come?" and "What did I do?" and "Is this real?"

Indeed, pain demands to be felt, in more ways than one.

But I also have something else. Something stronger than the two-pill solution every five hours. It's what has carried me these past few days and something I never expected.

It's the wishes.

They came from all over. Simple messages wishing me strength. Detailed prayers asking for healing. People pledging to do good things in the name of my complete recovery. They were texted, emailed, posted, and tweeted. Dinners were taken care of. Playdates were organized for my kids. And through it all, there was a steady stream of good wishes and hopes.

It was more than a simple gesture. It was magic.

Because with each wish that my husband read to me, each text that blew up my phone, each post on Facebook, each tweet—I felt myself getting better. It was as tangible as the two little white pills every five hours. I had never experienced anything quite like it. It was a million hands holding mine, carrying me, taking a bit of the pain away with each simple get-well message.

At the beginning of this journey, I was adamant about going it alone. Friends volunteered to accompany me to MRIs and biopsies and surgical consults, and I always said no. Alone, I was strong. I had to suck it up, face the music. Not having a shoulder to lean on meant that I would have to stand tall.

But now, after everything, it is all those wishes and prayers that have kept me standing. Those simple phone calls and quick notes have helped me in more ways than those two white pills. Those tweets have made me smile and laugh during ridiculously bad days, jump-starting my soul and my mind.

It's a bit clichéd to say I am grateful. So typical to say I am blessed. But that is what I am.

Grateful. Blessed. Preposterously lucky.
And I'm stronger each day.
Carried on the shoulders of wishes.

Side Effects

In the game of cancer defense, it's all about side effects. They were always there in the background, but now that the offensive season of surgery and recovery is over and the remaining pill-popping battle is more passive, everything seems to be a side effect.

WELL-MEANING FRIEND: You've put on some weight. You should tell your doctor.

ME: No. I actually ate an entire Duncan Hines cake by myself.

WELL-MEANING FRIEND: No. Weight gain is a side effect. You should tell your doctor.

ME: Did you just hear what I said? The *entire* cake. By myself.

WELL-MEANING FRIEND: You should tell your doctor.

ME: *(sigh)*

Or moodiness. That's a big one. I get angry at anyone and it's automatically chalked up to "side effects."

ANNOYING FRIEND: You know you're being snappy. That's a side effect.

ME: I think it's a side effect of you being an asshole.

ANNOYING FRIEND: No. You should tell your doctor.

ME: Tell my doctor that you're an asshole?

ANNOYING FRIEND: See? You're moody.

ME: *(sigh)*

You can't really win.

I mean, granted, there are a lot of side effects to the drugs I am taking. I'm exhausted all the time. Not just tired, by the way. Jet-lag tired. Like, if given the opportunity, I could sleep standing up. Which is kind of funny because the initial side effect of finding out you have cancer is, well, insomnia. Maybe I'm just making up for those months of sleepless nights with these current days of fatigue.

Then there's the nausea. Yes, it's a side effect, but I can rationalize that one away. I never had morning sickness when I was pregnant, so I'm thinking this is karma rather than an actual side effect.

Another unfortunate side effect of getting breast cancer is that my breasts have suddenly moved into the public domain and are acceptable topics during polite dinner conversation. This side effect was unnerving the first time it happened.

MALE DINNER GUEST: So, how is reconstruction going? Are you excited?

ME: *(spitting up seltzer)* Seriously?!

MALE DINNER GUEST: I mean, you must be happy, right? Women kill for this surgery.

ME: Actually, I think it's the surgery that kills them.

MALE DINNER GUEST: You know, I hear moodiness is a side effect.

ME: *(sigh)*

Not only is everything currently a side effect of whatever drugs I am taking, but every physical ailment is cause for alarm. I find myself constantly saying that line from

Kindergarten Cop, "It's not a tumah," when I ask a friend if she has any spare Advil in her bag.

I shouldn't complain, though. After all, one of the biggest side effects, at least hopefully, is that there won't be any more cancer crossing over to other parts of my body. That's a side effect that weighed heavily against the nausea, the fatigue, the brain fog, and whatever other gems this lovely ride plans on giving me.

However, I've decided not to google the side effects. After all, just because it's listed on the bottle doesn't mean it's because of the pills.

I'm tired from staying up late.

I'm gaining weight because I'm not watching what I eat.

I'm moody because . . . well, because people are idiots.

Though my husband has pointed out that my sarcasm has improved tremendously.

I told him it's a side effect.

Being a Rizzo in a Patty Simcox World

In case you didn't notice the pink billboards all over the highway or the placards at the checkout counter in your local grocery store, it's October, and that means it's Breast Cancer Awareness Month.

I would say that it's hard to miss, even if you don't drive I-95 or buy food. Prescription bottles are sporting pink childproof caps, Facebook is offering a temporary "Go Pink!" profile picture, and breast cancer cheerleaders are on street corners everywhere, shouting cutesy sayings like "Save the Ta-Tas!" or worrisome statistics like "One in eight women will be diagnosed. Will that be you?"

The first time I really noticed Breast Cancer Awareness Month was in October 2014 when I was recovering from a bilateral mastectomy and a cancer diagnosis that had fast-tracked me into a whole new plane of existence and a new level of intolerance for all things pink and sparkly. Especially ribbons, which seemed to be sprouting off everyone's lapels like weeds. Suddenly, everywhere I went, I was a card-carrying member of the trendiest party in town that I never wanted an invite to.

The timing was just off.

I should have been warned not to go to a breast cancer store that October. Having spent the summer battling post-cancer depression, I was in no mood to speak to the perky, happy-go-lucky breast cancer survivor who was fitting me for a lymphedema sleeve, my latest go-to apparel for flying and working out. I should have been nicer to her, but I had just come from PT and wasn't buying in to her chipper attitude.

WELL-MEANING BREAST CENTER LADY: So what kind of cancer did you have?

ME: Breast. That's why I'm at the Breast Center.

WMBCL: Haha! I know! *(squeal)* I mean, what kind?

ME: The kind that you take your breasts off for.

WMBCL: Ooh. Yeah, that must be why you need this. *(holds out lovely, skin-colored arm stockings)*

ME: *(glares)*

WMBCL: And what's your treatment plan?

ME: Alcohol. Alcohol and chocolate. In large quantities.

WMBCL: I'm sure you're discussing it with your doctor. Is your doctor here at—

ME: I don't discuss anything with doctors. I'm against medicine. In fact, my husband did the surgery himself, with a coat hanger, some whiskey, and duct tape. Can I just have the f-ing sleeve, please?

WMBCL: . . . I'll get your size. Would you like the pink one?

It was like shooting a puppy.

The cheerleaders were everywhere that October. "Pink Day" at work was a slow kind of torture. Wearing all black, I walked into a sea of hot-pink shirts. When a friend of mine asked why I wasn't wearing pink, I told her I decided to come to work with fake breasts, weight gain, and depression. It was a much more realistic picture than a happy pink tee.

I wasn't exactly the most positive person to be around. In a sense, I was a Rizzo, angry and snarky and missing her period, fighting the Patty Simcoxes of the world as they celebrated and cheered on "awareness." I wanted to crawl into a hole. Maybe take some of them with me.

But my take on Breast Cancer Awareness Month has changed with time. As I dealt with all the side effects of my new reality, I made peace with the cheerleaders on the streets and the "Run for Cancer!" ads that showed up in my inbox on a daily basis. I was hardly grabbing the pom-poms, and my sarcasm hadn't dimmed, but I slowly opened up to the shirts, the sentiments, the understanding of the rah-rah in bringing awareness to the masses. I gave a speech. I shared my perspective. I convinced some people to get mammograms.

The fallacy of Breast Cancer Awareness Month is that it's only a month, while breast cancer is a 24/7, 365-day-a-year fight. Even so, for 31 days, the excitement of the cheerleaders, the chipper ribbon-wearers, and the pink lymphedema sleeve-sellers, as well as the ever-present pink hue, definitely bring breast cancer research to the forefront of the country's mind. It is validating. It's a communal nod to a disease that desperately needs a cure. And it reminds women to do whatever they can to take care of their breasts before their breasts conspire to kill them.

Having argued with doctors and rolled my eyes at naturopaths and oncologists alike, I'm clearly on the other side of Breast Cancer Awareness Month. While I'm still snarky about the pink, I've come a long way. Time does that, I suppose. So does a good prognosis.

It's been a few years since that first October, and this time I'll wear pink once this month and remind people about mammograms and statistics, and I'll smile at the pie-bakers and pink-frosted cupcakes in the bakery windows and high-five the runners in the "5K for the Cure" races. I'll even bite down on my sarcasm a bit. Because even Rizzo, with all her gruff and tough outer shell, was still a Pink Lady.

But keep your ribbons off my implants.

The Cancer Movie

In the movie in my mind, I am the valiant, card-carrying cancer warrior, a runner of marathons and wearer of pink. I carry a shield emblazoned with "I SURVIVED!" in huge letters as I cartwheel into oncology offices and sprinkle strength on other patients like fairy dust. I am the comforter of the lost and the downtrodden. For the ones who have lost hope or feel helpless, I am a rock.

I'm congratulated for maintaining a sense of humor in the face of adversity, a calm expression during moments of extreme pain. A role model and an inspiration, they call me.

It's a good movie, where I am the hero, and I win at everything. At life. At death. At any struggle. But it is, unfortunately, a movie.

Getting cancer is common these days. It's an epidemic. Fortunately, there are enough movie scripts for dealing with it that I already know how my days will play out. The familiar tropes pop up so often in my real life that I'm no longer surprised by their appearances. I just continue playing the role that I was thrown into. I know how to make everyone laugh at me. I know every breast joke. I've written my own stand-up routine. The one-liners and comebacks are right at my disposal. After all, I've been watching these tearjerker movies since *Terms of Endearment*, and *my* story has a happy ending. I'm not turning into the wind beneath anyone's wings so quickly.

But there is an unscripted part of cancer that I haven't found in movies or TV. It's the part that is debilitatingly real. It's that part that makes its appearance during sleepless nights and 2 a.m. phone calls to friends. It's the shameful, weak, pathetic part of the cancer warrior. The part that fears surgery. That is terrified of the drugs constantly coursing through her body. The part that wonders if all that's left is the cancer warrior. If that shield will forever be held up for everyone to see. If it will be the *only* thing they see. The part that worries that the pre-cancer person is gone, replaced by someone who looks like a hero but is really just a fragile, scared, wretched girl, looking for someone else to be the champion. Looking to be saved. Looking to get back to where she was before her life was turned upside down.

In short, a fake.

Pain doesn't always have a logical cause. For weeks, I felt the physical pain of surgery, recovery, and reconstruction. I took my meds and threw myself into distractions as my body healed. But as the physical pain subsided, something happened; I wasn't bouncing back. Instead, a cloud moved in, consuming my nights with a different pain. Guilt that maybe I brought this on myself. Shame that I couldn't just be happy that I was going to survive. Profound loss for the disaster that was my body, my mind, my soul.

I tried to intellectualize it. I knew that I was so lucky. It was only stage I. Some people with less-fortunate diagnoses would do anything to see that on a pathology report.

And yet. And yet.

Sometimes pain isn't logical.

There is no logic with this cancer thing. If left alone, it will kill you. If treated, it still kills you. At least a part of you. People who have been there have told me it gets better. Even with the years of medication and all the horrible side effects, they tell me I will get back to the old me.

I'd like to believe them.

Most people think I'm already there. They pack this experience up into a neat box with comments like "So you're done?" or "So you must feel great! You're done!"

And I guess, for everyone, I am. I'm back. I'm smiling. I'm telling jokes. I'm the warrior. A survivor.

But all I am truly grateful for, truth be told, is that they can't see me at 2 a.m.

Can't see me at all.

Until my movie starts again the next day.

Jack Bauer Fixes Everything

"You need some serious distractions."

Those were the wise words of my older sister on the phone when I shared my worries and concerns while I was recovering from the third reconstruction surgery. Kind of ironic, because distractibility is pretty much my calling card. You'd think I'd have it down to a science.

But clearly I needed a nudge and a reminder that instead of trolling the internet for random articles and research studies with some vague connection to myself, I needed to just find something mindless to keep my brain occupied (ironic as that might seem).

Enter Jack Bauer.

I was a huge *24* fan back in the day, though I came to it a bit late. While everyone on the planet was watching season 6, I was catching up by watching seasons 1–5 on DVD. Watching those shows was probably the closest thing I've ever had to a serious addiction. It was like cocaine. I could not stop. I considered taking off work for a week just to finish all the seasons. I was up until 3 a.m. telling myself,

"Just one more episode." Or worse, "I'll just watch the first ten minutes."

I cried when the series ended and went into some serious withdrawal.

I tried *Homeland*. Tried every *24* wannabe. But I missed Jack.

And then Jack was back with *24: Live Another Day*. Amazing!

Of course, as fate would have it, that was the year I was diagnosed with cancer , and I couldn't watch it. Missed the first seven episodes. While Jack was saving London, I was working on saving myself. Go figure.

So when my sister reminded me to find a distraction, I knew it was time to find Jack again. And there he was, waiting for me on Hulu and Fox online.

Throwing myself back into *24* was the best thing I could have done. Nothing puts pain in perspective more than watching Jack torture a member of some splinter-cell terrorist group. Nothing is better than watching a show that is as gripping as it is ridiculous. And nothing, really, can make me happier than hearing that oh-so-familiar exclamation: "Dammit, Chloe!"

I spent an afternoon catching up with Jack and watching him save London against all odds. Watched as the terrorists got the upper hand over and over. Watched as he tortured a nine-fingered villain. Watched as the good guys were caught and tortured some more. Watched as Jack miraculously recovered from gunshot wounds and easily drove through London's streets with his damaged arm.

So I know. It's fiction. Serious fiction. But still, there was something in the fiction that gave me a bit more courage, a bit more strength to deal with my own insane circumstances.

Interestingly, right before I went into the mastectomy surgery, my husband recorded me. I was already on another planet, hopped up on drugs and not completely coherent, but smiling and laughing. He knew I wasn't going to remember anything. And I didn't. When I watched the embarrassing recording a few days later (which will *never* be on YouTube, by the way), I was surprised that for some inexplicable reason, as I was wheeled into the OR, I called out, "Dammit, Chloe! You were supposed to save me!"

I'm not really sure why I said that. I hadn't thought about Jack Bauer for a while, and then right there, in the middle of everything, I remembered him.

I think it explains why we need fiction. When reality is too much to bear, when walls are collapsing, it is the fictional heroes who come to our rescue. They are the books we read to escape, the shows we throw ourselves into, and the movies that transport us. The hero we conjure at our moments of crisis, or even joy, changes depending on the situation. Movie lines become part of our conversations; the mannerisms we mimic from the characters of our youth return on call. Those characters stand around us like specters. They hold our hands and make us laugh, sprinkling our difficult realities with moments of fiction.

Jack Bauer didn't save me from surgery. But he saved me after. In the midst of chaos and pain and depression, I was off saving London. For six hours, I wasn't thinking about cancer or pathology. I was just having a good time, Percocets and all.

I was freakin' Jack Bauer.

And Jack Bauer always saves the world.

Not bad for a little distraction.

The Things They Brought

They brought cards and balloons and bouquets of flowers. Tulips and sunflowers that brightened the grayness of the hospital room. They brought magazines and distractions and sock monkeys in varying shades of pink. They brought chocolate and cookies and homemade cakes.

They brought things I didn't realize I needed. A closet of button-down shirts and soft pajamas. Cotton robes and warm socks. They brought cold drinks to soothe my sore throat and blankets to wrap up in while I sat in one place. They brought pillows. Someone brought a gripper to reach things while my arms refused to work the way they used to. Someone offered to wash my hair.

They brought things that defined them and our relationships. They brought movies to watch, books to read, and season 1 of Sherlock. They brought audiobooks to listen to when it was impossible to focus. They brought notebooks to write in and even a poster with corny platitudes. They brought playlists on Spotify and flash drives of music.

They brought food. Daily. They brought ziti and chicken with rice. Brownies and cookies and coffee cakes. They brought hamburgers and roasts. French fries and pizzas. They brought macaroni and cheese and quiche. They brought challah and rolls, fish and rice. Lasagna and chocolate. They brought a month's supply of frozen soups. They felt bad that they couldn't bring more.

They brought love and good wishes and hopes and fears. They brought compliments and blessings, strength and compassion. They brought humor and tears. They brought light.

They brought stories. Their own and their friends'. Stories of survival. Stories of the fortunate. They brought tips and coping skills. They brought anecdotes and articles. They brought apologies and regrets that they couldn't do more. They brought jokes and laughter.

They brought help in ways I never expected. They brought family to and from the airport. They drove my children to school and brought them home again. They went shopping and called from wherever they were, asking if I needed anything. They reached out.

They defined themselves and the community. They brought whatever they could to shield me from fear and pain. They took my hand even when I wasn't reaching for it. They pulled me out of darkness and showered me with light. Their blessings danced in front of me and lifted me up.

They brought good wishes even though I insisted I was fine.

They waited with me.

They brought me hope.

They brought so much that when I started writing thank-you cards, I could only cry, amazed by who they became, by who they are. Amazed that they chose me to embrace and envelop with undeserved love.

They brought themselves. They brought their hearts.

And they saved me.

"I Didn't Want to Bother You"

Ahem.

Is this thing on? Good. Listen up.

Lesson of the day: bother them.

I learned a great deal over these past years, and one of the important takeaways from my experience is that I will never tell a friend in need that "I didn't want to bother" her. I heard those words many times from friends who didn't call, or email, or try to reach out to me when I was going through a rather difficult time. I would run into someone on the street, and their first response would be, "Oh. I didn't call you because I didn't want to bother you." Or, "I didn't want to bother you. I figured you had so much going on."

Unfortunately, I'm an English teacher. My superpower is in subtext.

"I didn't want to bother you" means that you didn't want to bother. Sometimes it means that you really just don't give a crap, but usually it means that the thought of making a phone call is so difficult that you'd rather hide behind an excuse of "I'm staying out of your way." It's a convenient rationalization. It's a way to convince yourself that you are helping someone by doing absolutely nothing. It isn't that you didn't want to bother me, it's that you didn't want to bother yourself.

Maybe you didn't know what to say. Maybe you felt out of place. But friendship and compassion are not about "not bothering." They are about knowing how to bother someone. They're about knowing when to step up.

I had friends who sent me cards. Friends who called and FaceTimed. I had one friend who left a message on my phone once a week, saying "You don't have to call me back, but I want you to know that I am thinking of you and you can call me whenever." I had friends who showed up at my door and just visited. I had friends. I had friends that emailed me. The phone call was too difficult, and I get that. But they still reached out. They helped.

They didn't hide behind "not bothering" me.

Years ago, a friend of mine lost a child in a tragic accident. I wasn't around when the tragedy took place, and so I knew that I would have to call her. I couldn't do it. I didn't know what to say. I didn't know how she would react. I couldn't even imagine the pain and horror that she was going through. But I also knew that I had no choice. If she was my friend, my discomfort was meaningless compared to her experience. It would be a terrible, horrible phone call, but it was a call I needed to make.

So I called her. And we cried. And she spoke to me. And she thanked me. She needed that support, as lame and ineffective as it probably was. Truth is, I could easily have told her that I didn't want to bother her and avoided that uncomfortable, inconvenient, sad phone call. I am sure there were many other people who did just that.

If you find yourself saying "I didn't want to bother you," I guarantee that you don't really mean it. You are trying to find an excuse to not bother yourself, assuaging your guilt because you can't think of something to say.

Say something. If you can't, then send a card. Write an email. And if for some reason you really think you might be bothering—take the risk. Make a call.

Lesson learned.

Speech over.

Mastectomy Mikvah

I was preparing to go to the mikvah.
I went through the laundry list of items to check:
My nails.
My ears.
My toes.
Is my hair combed?
Did I floss?
The mikvah is the place I go every month after my period ends. It's a ritualistic bath—a place where I go in clean, with no dirt or impurity—to dunk in the waters and then return to my husband, who has been off-limits for the week leading up to my immersion. It's a process I have followed since I was married, so it was familiar. A part of my life. I knew what to do and could do it by rote.

Besides, even with the diligence of my mental checklist, the mikvah lady would always double-check, going through her mantra while half listening for my reply or random nods. Of course I did everything. I've been doing it for years.

But the mikvah visit after my bilateral mastectomy was completely new. Even though I had that list running through my head, I couldn't focus. There were new items to check. Will I be allowed to go under water with the surgical glue still attached to my skin? Will I get an infection from the water? The drains are out, the scabs are soft—is that okay? I had spoken to the rabbi for guidance, but the enormity of what I was doing weighed heavily. Further, the idea of going into the mikvah and having the attendant watch me was terrifying. What subtle judgment would she make on seeing the scars that covered my chest, seeing my bruised and battered body still healing from the ten-hour surgery weeks before? Would she look at me with pity ("Oh. I'm so sorry you have cancer"), or would it be disgust? I imagined the "oh my God, that's horrible" look on her face upon seeing my Frankenstein-esque chest.

And what would I think, going into the waters? I had been taught to cross my arms in front of me as I said the blessing before I dipped in the "purifying" waters. But what was I covering now? Should I even do that? And how could I look at these waters as purifying ever again? The anticipation of mikvah, the romance of coming home after two weeks of separation from my husband was, I felt, permanently marred.

I prepared in the tiny room and dreaded pressing the call button that would indicate my readiness to dip. I wasn't ready. I was far from ready. I wasn't just checking my nails and combing my hair. I was looking in the mirror at a reflection that I did not recognize. There was no beauty in what I saw. No "you're so strong" image. I was a disaster. And I was about to put that disaster on display.

If I expected some compassion, I was mistaken. The attendant simply looked away from me—confirming my assumptions. She went through the list and ignored my numb responses. But then she asked pointedly about the black glue that still held tight. Did I have stitches? She wasn't sure if it was allowed. I told her I spoke to the rabbi, but she commented, offhandedly, "Well, if you say so," as if I was doing something so wrong. As if this wasn't the hardest thing ever. As if I had not silently wished that the rabbi had said no, you can't go, so that I could delay this horrible experience.

I stepped into the water, the first time in a long time, thinking that maybe if the cancer didn't kill me, the infection from the mikvah might. I turned around and faced the wall. The mikvah lady was behind me. I realized that crossing my arms in front of me wasn't even possible. My fear of touching the scars there made it impossible, and all I thought about was how much worse that would be when I came home to a husband who longed for that touch.

I said the blessing and dunked. The attendant announced that the process was "kosher"—everything was good. But the announcement stung. I wasn't kosher. I half laughed to myself that I could never be a sacrifice. I was too maimed.

As I emerged, the attendant held up a towel for me. She held it above her eyes—a practice that I knew was just for privacy—but at that moment, I believed it was shielding her from catching a glimpse of me. I didn't feel pure or holy. I was Grendel, the monster coming out of the depths into the mead hall where everyone is joyous and celebrating, coming to destroy that peace and light.

I went back into the small preparation room, dried off, and got dressed without looking at the mirror. I was supposed to be grateful. I was supposed to be thankful to God that I was alive. That I was going to be "fine." That I was just going to go on with my day-to-day, and this moment would be just a blip on the screen. But in that room, in that place where I was supposed to spiritually connect to myself, to God, to my husband—I was empty, certain I would never be complete again, positive that my "new normal" would never be anything remotely normal again.

But I had to walk out. I had to drive home. And so I splashed water on my face, held up my head, smiled at the attendant as I paid the fee, and got in my car.

I live five minutes from the mikvah.
It took me an hour to get home.

Doing Drugs

I have become an old woman.

I'm not talking about gray hair, or creaking bones, or any of that standard stuff. (Though I'm getting those as well.) No, this kind of aging is the stereotypical old-woman-in-a-home thing.

I became a pill-popping, coughing, miserable mess.

It's one thing to get the flu. But getting the flu on top of getting cancer just pisses me off. I mean, seriously? Because if you've ever had the flu, you know that you feel like dying. And if you've ever had cancer, you know that you might legitimately *be* dying. Wrap those two together, and you might as well just be knocking on the gates.

All I was thinking was "Great. So cancer didn't kill me, but pneumonia will."

There is tremendous irony at play in the world.

Apparently, as my oncologist pointed out to me as I was hacking up a lung, the medicine that I am on could weaken my immune system. That translates into "your cold is my pneumonia."

Fun.

So that aside, I was suddenly prescribed a whole host of pills and medications that became part of my daily regimen for ten days. You might not think that's such a big deal, but when one of the pills was roughly the size of a healthy newborn, I started to wonder if the drug companies had lost their collective minds and if maybe, just maybe, they were out to kill me. But I took that mother of a pill. Every morning and every night. Even though I was still coughing so much that I could no longer speak.

And then came the prednisone.

If you aren't familiar with that happy pill, let me spell it out for you. Some people have become psychotic taking it. Some people have become violent. Some people have driven cars off cliffs because of prednisone. But that didn't concern me. High on my list of concerns was the side effect written right under the psychotic break: "May cause weight gain."

Of course. Why not?

Between the prednisone, the Augmentin, the tamoxifen, the Lexapro, the Nyquil, the Sudafed, the Advil, and the cough drops, I needed one of those pill cases my grandmother used to have with the days of the week printed on top.

I told my doctor I was considering becoming a meth addict because at least I would lose weight. And if I was going to become a raving homicidal maniac, at least I'd look good in court.

Oncologists, I've discovered, need to work on their humor. Sigh.

I shouldn't complain. Though it's true, there are probably more drugs in my blood than platelets, and I did try to kill my husband in his sleep because he put the "wrong" sheets on the bed (he forgave me—prednisone perk), at least my coughing has stopped and I have no fever.

Also, it isn't like it's cancer or anything.

That would be much worse.

Happy Birthday Again

Lately, the problem with birthdays is that they are just so . . . yearly.

I always get philosophical on my birthday. You know, it's another year on the planet. It's a time to look back at everything I did or did not accomplish over the year. I'm lucky that I have a June birthday. It's six months after New Year's, and I get a chance to reassess those failed resolutions from January. It's like the midterm exam, and I get to buy myself new notebooks and pencils for the second term.

Last year, I spent my birthday recovering from a bilateral mastectomy. On a scale of one to ten, I would place that birthday squarely in the "one" category. The only reason I wouldn't make it a total zero is because, at the very least, I had some serious drugs to keep me on planet happy and was pretty busy rewatching every season of *24*.

And looking back at these past few weeks, this year's birthday is shaping up to be one of those real walking-on-the-beach, philosophical, what-is-the-meaning-of-life sort of days.

But I'm not falling into that trap again. No, siree.

Here is how I am spending my birthday this year:

I'm going to go see some mindless end-of-the-world destruction flick, and I'm going to eat a jumbo bag of popcorn and drink a Coke. The real stuff, mind you. None of that Coke Zero crap. I'm going for full-out calories and sugar. I'm even going to get ice cream after and maybe take a walk on the beach.

I'm going to get home and binge-watch some mindless Netflix series.

I'm going to drink wine and toast to a summer of books, beaches, and tequila.

I'm going to kiss my kids goodnight, snuggle them in their covers, and thank God that I have another year. Another year to get pissed off, to cry, to laugh, to get frustrated, and to get inspired. Another year to celebrate my kids' birthdays. To watch them struggle and succeed. To hear them complain about having nothing to eat in front of a fridge full of food. To hear their door slam when I take their phones away, or ground them. To hear them laugh and play in the yard with their friends.

I'm going to hang out with my husband and lie out in the backyard, taking advantage of the last breezy evenings before summer really kicks in. I'm going to hold hands and find fireflies and toast the midnight when the day ends.

It's my birthday. And I'm done with the philosophy and the introspection. Done with the midterm "where is my life going?" woes. I'm metaphorically switching schools this year. Moving from the Ivy Leagues to the party schools. Cornell to UC Santa Cruz.

Because really, birthdays should be about blessings and wishes.

And I've definitely had a year full of those, regardless of the insanity that permeated the year.

So pass the cake. I've got some candles to blow out.

There Are No Lessons Here

It's another October, so my newsfeed and emails are once again filled with pink ribbons and breast cancer fundraisers. This time, it's two years since my surgery. It's the time of year I've finally grown comfortable with and can laugh about without being triggered. I even started participating in "Pink Day" with an actual pink shirt. But I still bristle at the questions I sometimes get about how I've changed. What changes have I made in my life? What have I learned? Am I eating more kale?

I know everyone wants to hear them. The Oprah or Dr. Phil segment where someone tearfully extols some valuable life lessons that hardship has taught. Or the epiphany where everything is wrapped up in a convenient teachable moment and distilled into a TED Talk or a three-minute YouTube clip.

Truth is, there are no lessons here. If anything, my experience probably made me more cynical and short-tempered. I lost patience for the inane conversations I used to engage in, and I'm way more judgmental of people who can't handle

118

the simplest situations. I wouldn't call those lessons as much as I'd call them side effects.

My husband and I recently had a year-in-review conversation when we went over everything that has been happening in our lives and the lives of our children. And we agreed that there is no silver lining anywhere. You try to find it, but the bottom line is that when trouble hits, it hits. When things suck, they suck. There are no blessings to find when you're waiting for MRI results. No "we're so lucky" while waiting on a bone scan. Nothing silvery and glittering when your twelve-year-old is hit with theological questions most people don't grapple with until they're forty.

So no, Virginia, there are no lessons here to take away and impart on those more fortunate.

But we did somehow win some consolation prizes in the aftermath of chaos. Whenever you go through a painful situation or a difficult time, as unfair as the world seems, you also gain a unique look into the best that people can be. You witness your children stepping it up, behaving the way you hope they will behave as adults. You see a community that wants to help. Friends who want to join you.

And you meet new people, deeper people. You develop richer friendships. I called a friend of mine who I met through breast cancer and told her that she was my silver lining. I also told her it probably isn't a compliment that she meets her best friends when they're in crisis, but whatever. It works. Kind of like a twisted Stockholm syndrome. Without the Stockholm. Or the syndrome.

It's easy to wax poetic about pain and suffering. It's easy to slap on a pink ribbon and "Go Pink!" for cancer. Easy to hashtag posts with #blessed and #grateful and #savethetatas. Even though a part of me knocks it a bit (see "becoming cynical" above), I get that it serves a larger purpose of spreading awareness, and hope, and love. And I've gotten a lot better at joining that parade.

But the lessons learned can't be disseminated through hashtags and tweets or addressed in a five-second sound bite at the local 5K. I think, in learning that there are no lessons, we've just moved forward from that time. Learning, maybe, that nothing is ever set in stone, including the lessons you think you learned.

CAREGIVER

When I got the call that the MRI showed a large area of cells that probably hid cancer (Surprise! It did.), it was the last day of Passover. A year to the day from that call, my youngest son had a seizure while sitting on our couch, surrounded by friends from our community who'd come to hang out. I sat in the ER with the tech, watching the CT scan. I saw the large circle that immediately appeared on his brain image and knew it couldn't be good.

At the time, I was on tamoxifen. I was in the middle of reconstruction surgery. In fact, I had one last surgery scheduled for the week after the holiday.

Everything stopped.

I canceled my upcoming surgery. I stopped taking the tamoxifen. I put my health aside and focused solely on him.

That moment launched me into a new world that I didn't know existed.

At first, we were relieved to find out the tumor was benign. It was only after the surgery that we understood what a "benign" brain tumor looked like. We thought they would remove the tumor and we would all live happily ever after. But that wasn't the case.

The world of pediatric low-grade gliomas is a world that doesn't seem to end. For three years, we tried to balance the side effects from my son's surgery and help him manage his "new normal." We were told that the tumor would never come back and that we were in the clear.

But three years later, we had a scan that not only showed progression but indicated that the tumor had spread to the spine and to different areas of my son's brain. The news would send us from the neuro floor to the oncology ward, where we researched treatments and side effects and options for halting the spread of the tumors. When I called my husband to let him know about the scan, he crashed his car into a tree, devastated by the unexpected return of what was supposed to be an indolent tumor.

The relapse exploded on my family—sending us right back to that day of his first seizure. It has kept us captive, slaves to slowly changing scans and second opinions and researching treatment options that last years, not months. It taught us to make peace with the word "stable" when what we wanted was "NED" or "No Evidence of Disease." We learned how hard it is to fight slow-growing tumors, tumors that are passive-aggressive. Tumors that don't behave the way they're supposed to.

I was the medical person, in charge of out-of-state doctor visits to top oncologists and neurologists, making sure we did everything we could. I became the caretaker to everyone, managing my family's fears and concerns while trying to keep my own in check. I learned to navigate the world of pediatric brain tumors, networking with physicians, researchers, foundations, and other families who have been touched by this disease.

I didn't want my identity as a cancer mom any more than I wanted my son to be the brain tumor kid, but sometimes, I guess we don't always get to choose our roles.

Getting the Wind Knocked Out of Me

When I was thirteen, I was kicked in the solar plexus. It was during a karate class in seventh grade, and the girl I was sparring with delivered the roundhouse kick a bit stronger and faster than we were supposed to. It knocked me down and I gasped for breath, feeling like I had been shot. The sensei came over to me and reprimanded my partner and he then explained to me that I had "gotten the wind knocked out of me."

And he was right. Quite literally, in fact. I couldn't breathe.

But he also told me to lift my hands over my head and take huge gulps of air, even though it was difficult. I did what he said, and soon enough, the pain went away, I was breathing normally, and I could continue with the class. No bruise. No residual effects. No broken ribs. I stepped back in the ring and continued to spar.

Hearing that your son has a brain tumor knocks the wind out of you in a completely different way. I didn't fall to the floor and clutch at my chest. I wasn't gasping for air.

But I felt that sharp stab of pain, that helpless "I think I might die" feeling. It was as real as if I had been punched in the chest. Suddenly I was reeling, and the more the doctors repeated the findings, the further away from reality I felt.

It could not be true. There's no way. Not now. Not him. I just spent a whole year telling my son that there was no way he could catch cancer. That what happened to me would never happen to him. And there I was, in the ER on a Friday, getting called out as a liar. Because suddenly, the boy who should never have gotten a tumor had one.

I was hit again and again that evening. Watching him in an MRI machine. Watching him get a CAT scan, get an EEG, get gifts from well-intentioned nurses and friends. Each blow knocked me down, knocked me to the floor like that roundhouse kick in seventh grade, knocked me into a reality I was not prepared to face.

My sensei was right, though. I had to breathe. So I concentrated on that. Just inhaling deeply, lifting my arms up over my head, and breathing through everything that happened that weekend. Breathing through the blows as they came again and again. It was like childbirth. All I had to do was get over that jolt. Get my wind back. Breathe deeply and fully so I could stand.

We were guided by top neurologists and neurosurgeons. We surrounded ourselves with professionals. I read medical journals written in a language that was clearly English, but the vocabulary was so over my head that, like a child, I just looked at the pictures. I compared them to my son's MRI images, trying to get some idea of what we were in for. We were enveloped by friends and family and told over and over again to just breathe. Just take steps. Stop thinking about worst-case scenarios. Trust the doctors. Trust the surgeons. Trust in God.

And while we were getting the wind knocked out of us, we discovered we weren't alone. Thousands of people joined us to pray for our son. To do good deeds. To respond to this terrible blow by creating more light in the world. While we sat in that pediatric surgical waiting room, we read post after post from strangers and friends alike. Posts that reminded us to breathe and take big gulps of air. Posts telling us that as worried as we were, as terrifying as the situation was, we would be okay. My son would be okay.

Every step was difficult. Every "what if" debilitating. But he made it through. He opened his eyes after that grueling eight-hour surgery and asked for a cup of water. He even cracked a joke that night in the ICU. As we crossed each hurdle, we shared it with the people who carried us through. "He woke up!" "He spoke!" "He ate food!" Each tiny step was another deep breath that lessened the pain and the worry. It allowed us to stand up again. Get our wind back.

A friend asked me how I could deal with this so soon after my own health issues last year. I guess I learned how back in seventh grade. When you get kicked in the chest, when the wind gets knocked out of you, you just breathe.

And then you step back into the ring.

Healing

When my son was diagnosed with a brain tumor, my husband and I focused on treating him and getting him better. He needed tests—MRIs, EEGs, evaluations—and he needed surgery. I was suddenly introduced to new words I had never heard before and new worlds that had little to do with my previous day-to-day. I was monitoring medications and side effects, watching for seizures, changing my son's diet, and reading up on everything I could get my hands on regarding his tumor, his condition, his prognosis. Every little concern prompted a call to one of his many doctors and a follow-up Google search just to double-check the doctor's advice.

And so we worked on healing him. We wanted everything to go back to normal. He would have surgery and return to school and we would all live many, many more years. Happily ever after.

But we soon learned that brain surgery is a little more complicated than that. And you can't mess around in someone's head and expect everything to be the same as it was before. We also didn't consider the repercussions for our son and what going through this experience would mean to him. We worried. All the time. When he was going to a friend's house or riding a scooter. At school, he wasn't getting back into the swing of things. Subjects he used to find easy were suddenly challenging. The schoolwork was taking him longer. His memory was shot. His handwriting changed. He was angry and miserable, and we just smiled, staying positive as we shuttled him to OT and tutors and follow-up MRIs and doctors.

We thought we were healing him.

It took an organization to show us that we had forgotten the missing piece in my son's—and my family's—healing.

An organization dedicated to supporting children and families in crisis and through illness had been by our side since my son's original diagnosis. On one particularly difficult day, when I was having a meltdown almost as large as my son's, the regional director suggested I send my son on a trip to Orlando. Through another organization called Ohr Meir, kids from all over the country with life-threatening illnesses come together for a four-day, action-packed, distraction-laden trip to the theme parks and attractions in Orlando.

I was hesitant.

For starters, my son no longer had a life-threatening illness. His tumor was benign. He didn't need chemo or radiation. I didn't want to identify him as a "sick kid." Though we knew it would be a few years before we were totally in the clear, his prognosis was good. Besides, I didn't think he'd even want to go. This is a kid that doesn't even go to birthday parties. He'd never slept over at a friend's house. There was no way he would want to be away from us for four days, Disney notwithstanding.

I missed the whole point, though.

This wasn't a trip about Disney. It was about meeting other kids who get how awful the IV team at the hospital can be. It was about meeting kids who intimately know what the inside of an MRI is like and how bad hospital food can really get. It was meeting kids who take medicine all the time, who miss school for doctor visits and tests. It was meeting kids who have parents who are always worried and teachers who don't understand their new limitations. It was meeting kids who also had brain tumors and went through surgery. And more importantly, it was being in a place where, for four days, he didn't have to think about all that.

He jumped at the chance.

I didn't realize how crucial this trip was for my son's healing. I thought, "Sure! Trip to Disney! Everyone loves Disney!"

I had no clue. I watched the transformation in the pictures that were updated on Snapchat, Instagram, Facebook, and WhatsApp by the overly caffeinated and highly energetic staff. Every second of the day was focused on keeping these kids away from their various diagnoses and ailments, focusing instead on just having fun. But I really didn't get it until my older son, looking at his younger brother in the pictures on my phone, said, "Wow! He's smiling! He never smiles like that!"

It was true. I hadn't even noticed it, but over the previous five months, he had lost that smile. It was forced in pictures and never came easy. Looking at the pictures that flooded my phone, I saw my son happy, for the first time in a long time. He wasn't thinking about the upcoming PET scan or the forty-eight-hour EEG that the neurologist had suggested offhandedly at the last visit like it was no big deal. I saw him being a kid. Being happy. Running around without neurotic parents or demanding teachers or meddlesome residents with their IVs and needles.

Healing is not just about the medicine. It is about happiness. My son might not be the same as he was before the surgery, but there is more to his life than catching up and staying ahead of seizures and tumors. Ohr Meir's amazing staff gave that gift to me. They gave that gift to him. They reminded me what my son truly needed in order to heal. He needed to be a kid. And we needed to remember what that looked like.

Becoming That Neurotic Mother

Having a kid who has brain surgery changes one's parenting. I went from someone who took her kid to the doctor once a year to someone who has an entire team to choose from when something goes wrong.

There's a person to call for every possible new symptom and every possible new worry. In some sense, it's comforting. But it has also turned me into one of those neurotic mothers I used to scoff at on the playground.

Once you've become everyone else's worst-case scenario, it's hard to separate the day-to-day childhood ailments with the looming "oh my God this could be the end" scenarios. My son gets a headache, and I'm running to the phone. He trips on the stairs, and I'm rushing to check his vision. He says he's tired, and I quickly check to see if he took his meds that morning. And if he did, I'm researching side effects on Google.

On the other side of the spectrum, I've lost the ability to empathize when other mothers bemoan their kid's colds. Or their sprained ankles. Or their root canals. I listen to them freaking out, and a part of me wants to just slap them and say, "Do you know who you are talking to?" Because as nerve racking as your kid's ten-minute adenoid procedure might have been, I have vivid memories of being the first person in the pediatric surgical waiting room and the very last, watching parents come in and sit for fifteen minutes until their doctors came out to tell them they could come and see their kid.

My husband and I waited ten hours.

It isn't fair of me, really. Because I also know that just as I am many people's horror story, I am also a lot of other people's best case. And so my neuroses over my kid's head-ache pale in comparison to their experiences. For instance, my son's roommate on the neurosurgery floor was moved to the oncology floor before we even knew his name.

It's all perspective. I can vaguely remember when my oldest daughter had to have a small mole removed from her scalp when she was three years old. My husband and I cried as they wheeled her into the operating room for a procedure that probably lasted the same amount of time it took us to walk back to our chairs. At the time, it was frightening. The anesthesia! The medication! The tiny scar on her perfect scalp!

And I guess, for us, it was the worst-case scenario in our young parental lives.

I try to think back to that moment when someone cries to me about their own worst cases. I have to remind myself that whatever it is that they are dealing with, as insignificant and trite as it seems to me, it is *their* worst nightmare. At the same time, I have to remember that my heightened state of alert is probably just as baffling to them. My worry over my son sleeping too long would more than likely be met with an exasperated, "Dude, be glad he's sleeping!" Most other parents wouldn't understand the all-too-tragic and dramatic scenarios that instantly run through my head and send me to DefCon 2.

So I respond to the frantic moms fretting over splinters and stitches the way I always do: "This must be very hard for you." Because if there is one thing I also know, it's that when you're in it, pain is pain. And a child's pain, anywhere on the scale, is everyone's worst case. It's everyone's pain.

But secretly, I want to slap them.

The Power of a Cape

A year and a half ago, I was waiting for biopsy results that would eventually land me in the hospital with a bilateral mastectomy and a newfound appreciation for pain medication. But way before all that, I was playing the waiting game, hoping it was nothing, sure it was something, terrified of what would happen. It was a Thursday, and I was shopping for costumes with my kids when I saw the Superman cape. It was only the cape, no other accessories. No muscle suit or tights. The store owner wanted twenty-five dollars for it—a little pricey for a cape with no accoutrements—but I didn't care. I told my husband, "That cape is mine."

I wore it in the store. I wore it on the way home (ignoring the rolling eyes of my kids), and I wore it on Monday, when the biopsy results came in and I knew things were going to get real. It was a silly gesture, but for some reason, I was transformed. My kids saw me in a cape, and I told them, "I'm actually a superhero." They shrugged and walked off. I pretended to fly around the house.

I went through a year of surgeries and medications, and somewhere along the line, I lost my cape. I looked for it in the kids' costume box, searched my closet, even posted a message on Facebook asking if anyone had borrowed it. To no avail. My cape just disappeared.

Not that I needed it. Not then.

The superhero status transferred to my son a year later. Diagnosed with a brain tumor, he was facing a long surgery, and who knew what else. He didn't need a cape, though. He got an Iron Man mask. A gift from the food market that we shop in every week. "He's our hero," the staff said to me. One of the nurses hung up a poster in his room, telling him he had joined the Avengers. And we all convinced him that the brain surgery gave him powers.

"If you find yourself understanding things quicker and noticing that you're smarter," I said to him, "don't worry. That's normal after brain surgery. It's just your brain getting bigger. Use your powers wisely."

There is something about a cape, about a mask, about an external, tangible symbol of strength and determination. It's a physical reminder that is much more powerful than a pink ribbon or a hashtag on Twitter. Simply put, it is the power of fictions to topple the bleak reality that life dishes out. More than an escape, more than just cosplay, it changes your persona. Put on a cape, and you are transformed. Invincible and brave, regardless of what Edna Mode says.

I recently needed my cape again. A year and a half after that first biopsy, I needed another one to check for possible uterine cancer. My husband and I kept it quiet this time, but I confessed to my doctor that I believed God was out to get me. That I was supposed to die. That this time, I wouldn't have to wait for results because I would never wake up from the anesthesia.

He gave me some Xanax; I considered finding a new doctor.

The night before the procedure, I didn't sleep. I googled my symptoms, and like with any decent Dr. Google consultation, confirmed the worst. At 3:30 a.m., though, annoyed with sitting around, I went into my closet and packed up my bag for the next day. A book. My phone charger. Socks. And then, right there, sitting on a shelf as if it somehow knew, was my long-lost cape.

And I was transformed.

I packed my cape. Folded it gently and put it in my bag. I wasn't going to wear it to the hospital (a stay in the psych ward probably would not be in the best interests of my family), but taking it along was empowering. My secret power, hidden away for only me to see. My fictions playing out as truth right there. So much better than reality. Far more effective than Xanax.

And after the waiting, this time, the biopsy was benign.

Call it what you will. Denial. Immaturity. Insanity. But then again, a year of breast cancer, brain tumors, and—plot twist!—possible uterine cancer is insanity on a whole different level. Given the choice, I'll side with superhero insanity any day.

My son has an MRI in two weeks. I told him not to worry. He's done it before. He'll be fine.

Plus, he comes from a family of Supers.

And he has my cape.

More Than a Hashtag

I didn't share your Facebook status, the "Share this with everyone!" directive notwithstanding. I ignored the attempted guilt trip as well. The baiting "Let's see who really cares" warning, complete with instructions on how to copy and paste the status in case anyone is new to the whole computer thing.

I didn't share it, even though I appreciated the multicolored hearts, the beautiful sentiments, the clever hashtags. I know that you are doing your part in raising awareness for whatever cause is currently trending. And I know the cause is worthy, judging from the number of likes and shares that your post generates. Your hashtags trend on Twitter, and for a small window of time, we are an online community of people dedicated to altruism and love and kindness.

All with a hashtag and a click of a button.

I don't know when the world started accepting that action and change require nothing more than two seconds of sharing. It's true, we are spreading awareness, getting the word out, letting people know we are outraged or compassionate, but we are lying to ourselves if we think that real change can be accomplished that way. Real change requires a commitment. It requires boots-on-the-ground action. It necessitates putting some teeth behind that hashtag, behind that status update.

As someone who has been touched by breast cancer and pediatric brain tumors, these posts tend to strike a nerve. I know the sentiment is coming from a pure place, but I also know there is so much that can be done beyond the copy-and-paste model that currently fills my newsfeed. Childhood cancer is on the rise. More women are being diagnosed with early-stage breast cancer than in previous years. Getting the word out about these diseases is important, but so is finding cures.

These cancer posts are particularly jarring. It's outrageous that even now there are still children dying from diseases that might be cured with proper funding for research. No amount of #f-cancer or #fightcancer postings will do anything. If we want to truly fight these devastating illnesses, we need to believe in science and fund the people who are working toward cures.

If you are moved enough to write a post on Facebook or Instagram, then move yourself to donate money to research. Write a status that says you gave money to help fight cancer. Send out a tweet with a link to places to donate. Bring awareness about cutting-edge research that needs funding so it can save lives, save families. Find foundations privately funded by families who have been shattered by these diseases and are working to ensure that no child has to endure what their child is going through. Actively take part in the greatest Kickstarter ever that's been running for years behind the scenes of every hashtag, meme, and status update but has somehow fallen behind the far easier "click and share" culture of publicly feeling good.

I am not a fundraiser. Thankfully, my son's tumor was benign and my breast cancer was caught at stage I. But so many others have seen the darker side, and that knowledge constantly reminds me that I have to do more than write 140 characters or slap a ribbon on my chest.

Keep your hearts and hashtags—awareness is important—but if you want to really do something, take up the fight. Next time you get a share on your timeline, next time you see a clever hashtag, donate to cancer research and share your action, not just your status.

Time is critical for some, but you can still make a difference.

Scientists are standing by.

Tears of Joy, Tears of Pain

It might just be a consequence of getting older. My kids are going off to college, to camp, to higher grades in high school. The family dynamic is shifting in subtle ways, and I am home in an empty house on more occasions than ever before.

It might also be a consequence of everyday life. I have had a few challenging years that have blessed me in the most backhanded way possible, reminding me on a daily basis to tell my kids I love them. To remember that we are all living on borrowed time and that at any second, the ground may come undone. It's the punch-in-the-face realization, the blessing one takes while yelling "Thank you, sir, may I have another!" to the great doler-outer of fortune and grace.

And so, I find myself crying more than I have in past years. Not just from pain, but from joy. The two have become intertwined, as I have come to recognize that the joys we have are tenuous. That moments need to be grasped, and captured, and branded into more than a Snapchat story that records them. But unfortunately, I can't take these smiles and joys and place them in bottles on my kitchen shelf to look at and save like a ceramic teapot collection. These joyous moments remind me of how time has incomprehensibly and silently sped up since my last birthday, since last year, since the last hour. And so I cry with the joy, and I cry with the pain, and my empty house echoes the same.

I know I am not unique in this. I remember seeing adults crying at weddings and telling myself that I would never be like that, and now, here I am falling apart over smiling pictures of my kids at camp and hiding in my closet so none of my other children will see.

They are tears of joy and tears of pain.

It's part of the blessings of hardship, or rather, of life. It is something I could never have comprehended at twenty-five, when my worst fear was that my then one-year-old daughter wouldn't get invited to a class birthday party. But now, having dipped my toe into a world of darkness, I know what possibilities lie ahead. I know what I've managed to escape, and my blessings are like shards of brilliant glass, reflecting light and brightness through dangerous spikes and splinters.

In a moment of quiet reflection, my ten-year-old son made a profound observation. He was commenting on how everyone always tells him he has challenges and that he overcomes them. "It isn't that I have challenges," he said, "it's that life is the challenge. Just living every day. Everyone has that, not just me. That's the real challenge."

I told my husband what he had said and remarked there is no way anyone would believe he actually said that. It seemed too perfect to come from the mouth of a kid his age. But now, looking at his smiling face in a picture, I realize that no one else could have said it quite so well. It resonates so clearly. The happy, the sad, the pain, the joy—it's the challenge of life, all-encompassing and overwhelming, never static and rarely quiet. How ironic that my youngest child understands that juxtaposition better than most adults.

My kids will make fun of my tears, and I'm glad. Most of them are still battling the simple obstacles. I know one day they will cry tears of joy, one day they will cry from pain, and one day, they will see the blessings in both.

For now, I need to just hang on to the blessings, shards and all, and embrace all the light I can find. Even if it means crying over camp pictures.

After all, these tears of pain are also tears of joy.

The Roller Coaster Moment

"I went on an upside down, backwards, crazy roller coaster!"

That was the message I got from my ten-year-old on WhatsApp. From my child, who had never gone on a roller coaster, who had always said he was scared of roller coasters, who I could not even convince to ride the kiddie coaster at the state fair.

That child went on an upside down, backwards, crazy roller coaster.

He was away at an overnight camp for kids with cancer and complex chronic illness. Going on the roller coaster might seem like a simple thing, something I shared with his siblings just to see their look of shock, but it has become something much greater.

It's easy to couch the experience in clichéd metaphor. For this child, the past year has been a figurative roller coaster with more drops than lifts. And the analogy works for anyone in a difficult situation, or for coping with the ordinary ups and downs of life. Sometimes you're going up, sometimes you're plummeting down, and sometimes you're just being flipped and dragged backwards through twists and turns and violent curves.

But going on this roller coaster was something completely different for my son. It took a great deal of coaxing on the part of the assistant head counselor, Tzvi Haber. An hour and a half of coaxing, to be specific. And there were tears, and begging, and cajoling on both sides. Like I said, my kid is not a thrill-seeker. His favorite activity prior to that moment was miniature golf.

I would never have forced the issue and would have just taken him to the go-carts. Tzvi, though, saw the moment as something much more important. He understood that this was something my son needed to do. He needed to face his fear, and he needed to do it himself.

I realized how far-reaching the experience was when I spoke to my kid again later that day. When he FaceTimed me and was absolutely beaming with a pride I have never seen on his face. He retold the story and then said he went on four more "big" coasters after that. I couldn't believe it.

Before we hung up, he said something that I found extraordinary.

"You know what?" he said, "Now I can do anything." And so I replied with the typical mom response of "That's right. You can do anything."

But he saw right through that and repeated, making sure I fully understood.

"No. Really. I can *really* do anything."

That was the moment, the moment when the roller coaster in his world started going up again, the moment that my ten-year-old understood the personal power he had inside. He wasn't passive; he was strong. He was confident. He could ride any coaster, figurative or literal, and come out triumphant.

"Kids need to get rid of the things they know they are afraid of," Tzvi said. It's true. My son is coming home from camp with the confidence he will need to face the year ahead. He's become accustomed to facing his fears of the unknown and dealing with challenges that seem insurmountable at times. The roller coaster moment when he faced down his fear and conquered something tangible—that moment will become his shield and sword for the challenges that lie ahead.

A simple roller coaster moment?

No, it was much more than that. It gave him power. It gave him courage. It gave him confidence.

It gave him the ability to jump on the next ride.

Two Years

Two years ago, my husband and I were sitting in a waiting room. We were the first people to show up at five in the morning, and we sat there all day watching other parents come and go. We were the last ones in the room when we finally left ten hours later.

It was a grueling day, made easier by the posts and messages we received as we waited for the neurosurgeon, Dr. Bhatia, to bring us news that our eight-year-old son was safely out of surgery and the brain tumor that had sideswiped my family was out. At the time, our concerns were acute—"Will he wake up?" "Will he be able to speak?" "Will he remember who we are?" As he recovered, those concerns were replaced by new ones—"Will he be the same?" "Will *we* ever be the same?"

We were given a simple plan: surgery, recovery, follow-up, happily ever after. Two years later, we are still following up. I recently told our surgeon that as simple as the postsurgical narrative seemed, it has been far more complex. We didn't realize that we would forever be altered. That from then on, whenever my son had a hangnail, we would give him a Band-Aid and then follow up with a Google search for "hangnails and brain tumor," just to make sure. We didn't realize the havoc medications and testing would create in our son's life. We didn't realize that calling a tumor benign when it's in a part of the brain that affects breathing and thinking is somewhat misleading. We didn't realize that nothing would ever be simple again.

We also didn't realize how lucky we were. It's hard to think that you're fortunate when your child is the one at the center of community prayers and meal trains. But two years ago, we had no clue how bad things could have been. As we met other families and saw worse scenarios play out, we guiltily embraced our fortune that our son was a frequent visitor of the neuro floor and not the oncology unit.

My brother, Rabbi Akiva Weiss, gave me a perfect analogy the other day as I was sharing our recent experiences in the "follow-up" stage of our seemingly never-ending saga. In the Harry Potter series, creatures called Thestrals are only visible to people who have seen death. In the third and fourth books, Harry is brought to Hogwarts by horseless carriage, but in the fifth book, after witnessing the death of a friend, Harry suddenly sees that the carriages were never horseless. The Thestrals pull the carriages up to the castle. Once you see these dark, disturbing, and magical creatures, you can't go back to seeing the horseless carriage. You're different, and you literally cannot see things the same way as others.

The Thestrals surround us constantly. They sit in waiting rooms with us and unfurl their wings around MRI machines and rest next to us during inpatient stays while we wait for more and more tests.

Two years ago, I didn't know anything about brain tumors or seizures. I didn't know anything about medical journals. I had never heard of the word "resection" before. I had no idea what was going to happen to my life, my son's life, and my family.

This morning, Facebook reminded me that two years ago, I was a different person. When I looked back on the memories that appeared in my feed, I was jolted back to that never-ending day when I was so naïve and uneducated. When I look back at that day, I sometimes think it wasn't real. Could that really have happened? Were my husband and I really sitting there all day? How did we even do that? I was reminded of the hundreds of emails and messages we received, people asking if they could help us, letting us know that they were with us.

Two years ago, we didn't realize that this would be the day we would always look back on—that we would always be counting onward from—as the day our definition of normal shifted permanently. We couldn't know how that one day would frame our every day, how it would lead us to new, deeper friendships, how it would lead us to get involved in organizations that help kids much sicker than our son ever was, how it would lead me to run a half-marathon.

Two years ago, we were just recovering from breast cancer, thinking that was the worst things would ever get.

Facebook just reminded me that two years ago, we were blessedly clueless, but also ridiculously blessed—and we continue to be so.

Two years and counting.

Survivor's Guilt

"Isn't your son doing well?"

I get this question all the time from well-meaning friends and concerned neighbors who see pictures of my son at a camp for kids with cancer and chronic medical conditions and wonder if there is something I am not telling them about my son's condition. It's hard to explain to them what that camp has done for my child and our family. It's one of those things that you need to experience to understand, and trust me, no one ever wants to pay for that steep entrance ticket.

At first, I didn't want to send him. I had conversations with various people after we received the invitation, and I was sure that I was going to be putting him in a situation where he didn't belong. I imagined a camp full of sick kids in treatment for cancer alongside my son, the kid recovering from a craniotomy to remove a tumor that wasn't going to kill him. I tried to look at his surgery like an appendectomy. We removed it. He recovered. Carry on.

But that first year after his surgery proved that philosophy wrong and unrealistic. School, which had been easy for him, was suddenly a nightmare. Everything was difficult. The medications he was taking affected his days and nights, and we were constantly taking him back to the doctors, sending him to the hospital for overnight tests, and waiting in trepidation for whatever the next MRI would reveal.

I missed so many days of work and was so distracted from my job that I was sometimes surprised when I saw a paycheck clear in my account. I was changed. I knew that no matter what, from the day of the surgery and onward, nothing would ever be the same. The invisible safety net that I had thought always surrounded my family had been snatched away, and so, even as my son improved, the worries never abated. I would walk to his room in the morning and hold my breath before opening the door, bracing myself in case I couldn't wake him. Fearing that maybe he had suffered a seizure in the night. Scared constantly by all the "what ifs."

And with those fatalistic and scary thoughts came the equally crippling fear that maybe I was crazy. Maybe I was making things larger than they were. I knew of kids in far worse situations. Kids who were not going to camp. Kids who spent months in the hospital in contrast with my son's sporadic nights there. It was difficult to balance—my happiness at his health and my awareness of the pain of others. As he grew stronger and healthier, my guilt grew. I was embarrassed by my worries, ashamed of my good fortune. And every time I tried to take stock, get grounded, and just close that door—go back to that time before my world changed—I couldn't. With every good report, I found myself waiting, always waiting, for whatever bad news would come next—news that I almost felt I deserved.

Perhaps he felt that. My son, the focus of my constant hovering and questions, must have sensed that when I kissed him goodnight, I cried in the shower later that evening. Sensed that I measured out my days since his surgery in moments and pieces instead of long years, always believing in the back of my mind that we were living on borrowed time.

People are so hardwired to be normal. To be just like everyone else. For my family, putting on that face of normalcy conflicted with the underlying sense that we were so far from it and would probably always be, try as we might to remedy it. It was isolating. We existed between two worlds. There was the world of pediatric brain tumors, where we were the best-case scenario and couldn't express our worries and fears to our new friends who had it so much worse. Then there was the friendly neighborhood world of skinned knees and strep throat, in which no one could fathom what our day-to-day was like. Somewhere, in that mix of emotions and stress and tears and relief, was my son. Struggling with his own fears, his own experience, and his own understanding, no matter how much I downplayed the next MRI, of what was at stake.

We watched him change that first year at camp, becoming more confident than we had ever seen. Mainly, he said he goes there and feels "normal," though ironically, if you saw him during the year, you would never imagine that he feels otherwise. My friends and neighbors would never believe it. But then, they aren't witness to the types of conversations he has with his counselors. They don't realize that his closest friends are much older than him. They can't understand that he went into that surgery as a child, and emerged more mature than some of the adults I know. He is light years beyond the typical eleven-year-old in terms of his experiences, his thoughts, and his ability to empathize with others.

I carry tremendous guilt when it comes to my son. Not just the survivor's guilt that any therapist would identify from a mile away, but guilt that I didn't do enough for him when I missed all the signs leading up to the discovery of this tumor, and guilt that I overcompensate now, being hypervigilant so I won't miss anything again. For a time, I beat myself up, convinced that his tumor was somehow my fault. (And for the record, one lovely woman was quick to point out that it probably *was* my fault because, after all, I allowed him to eat M&Ms. The red ones.) There's guilt when I look at pictures of him smiling, guilt that he *can* smile, and guilt that I can't send him away to a regular camp—not yet, not now—and guilt that he is getting better.

Why did I send my son? Because as crushing as my insecurities and my guilt sometimes become, I can't let my son be a victim of it. I give my son two weeks of joy, and I give my family two weeks to remember that he deserves it. His days that I carefully measure in appointments and symptoms are far better spent in shaving-cream fights and late-night dodgeball games. Much better spent on hammocks between trees, on boats, on ziplines, and on the shoulders of magical counselors who love him as fiercely as we do. Much better spent as an actual eleven-year-old.

Somewhere between closing the metaphorical door of any traumatic situation and getting sucked into the constant vortex of pain and victimhood, there's a middle place of relative contentment. Of just understanding that it is what it is. You can't keep defaulting to the worst-case scenario or you'll go crazy, but you can't ever really close the door. I'm not sure I've found that sweet spot yet, but maybe I'm getting a little closer to it. Initially, sending my son away made me think I was placing him squarely in the shadow of my fears and ensuring he would forever carry the victim card. Instead, it was the complete opposite. It freed him of it. I realized that first year that I really knew nothing. And even though the friends who ask me why I send my son there think they know what it's about, they can't possibly understand.

And hopefully, they never will.

Dear Blogger

Dear Blogger,

I read with great interest your recent post about why bad things happen to good people. I can't even begin to tell you how excited I was—the never-ending search for the answer to a question that has stumped philosophers and religious leaders for generations was finally going to be answered by someone from Jersey.

As a New Jersey native myself, I have to say, I am a bit disappointed. For while your response tries to be cogent and intelligent, it reads like a lower-level ninth-grade student's extra-credit philosophy paper. It isn't just the clichéd allusions and the undocumented ideas. After all, this is your own opinion masquerading as authority. No need to quote sources. I get it. What bothers me more is the sanctimonious nature of your piece. The way you assume so much, with no real understanding of the magnitude of your hollow epiphanies.

I'm going to give you a clue because you clearly don't have one. You are not in any position to tell anyone why anything happens in their lives. You might think that you have suffered and this somehow gives you the right to extol whatever lessons you found comfort in during your "journey" or your "experience," but it doesn't.

Because here's the deal: you don't know what someone else's suffering is. And I promise you this: even if you think you do, you still don't. No matter where you are on the scale of worst-case life experiences, I can point you in the direction of much harder, more painful stories that don't jive with your shallow, linear explanation of why bad things happen. Go hang out at St. Jude's for a day. Go visit a thirty-year-old woman in hospice. Even better, go hand out your article to the parents sitting near their child who's dying in a hospital bed. Go give it to kids sitting shiva for their parents. Laminate it for the world as a resource so that your answer can bring comfort to those who have suffered. And when you do, I suggest you wear Kevlar.

You know why? Because there's a reason generations of scholars and philosophers have grappled with this concept. There's a reason you can't look at people suffering and in good conscience say that they probably deserved it in some way. There's a reason it's wrong to simplify suffering, as you have done, in cutesy metaphors involving children and candy or teenagers and phones. And there's a reason we don't understand it. Because while you might think you have a clear vision of God and His ways, and you might really believe that you have the answers, those answers apply only to you and your situation. We all learn our own lessons as life gives us challenges. But the problem arises when you believe that since you have suffered through something, you now have the right to tell the world how they must feel—like you are an authority on the matter.

Therein is the problem. No one is ever an authority on someone else's pain. And no one is a speaker for God. Especially not someone banging out her philosophy on a laptop in Jersey. These questions require more depth.

More thought. And in general, more compassion and under-standing, which your limited experience prevents you from having.

Rule number one of writing is "Know your audience." If you're writing about why bad things happen to good people, you might want to rethink your tack a bit. I know too many good people—really good people—who have had too many bad things—really bad things—happen to them. Those peo-ple are reading your words. And they know a truth that you can't even begin to fathom in your sophomoric philosophy.

I will leave you with this. You don't know me, and that's good. I don't think we would have played together at the shore. But if you are going to put yourself in a public forum and throw your hat in with Maimonides, Job, and you know, God, I suggest you do your research. Because I am not one person here. I speak for a lot of people. This isn't a high-school philosophy class. There are no absolutes when it comes to pain. This is life, with all its complexities. With things we don't get. Things that can't be solved in a five-hundred-word post.

So stop pretending you can.

Lessons From a Hero

I've written about many of my son's experiences after his surgery to remove a brain tumor three years ago. Most of them are stories of healing and recovery—the stories about Disney World and the incredible people who helped us through the weeks and months and years after that day. But I have never written about the person at the center of his story, the man who literally saved our son. I have never written about Dr. Sanjiv Bhatia.

It's clichéd to call the man who saves your child "an angel." We handed our son over to this man—a stranger—and trusted everything he said, followed his orders, and prayed that he knew what he was doing. We were told that neurosurgeons are notorious for their inflated egos. They are at the top of the medical food chain, and people warned us not to expect much. "Expertise is more important than bedside manner," my friend told me.

Dr. Bhatia had both. On the first day we met him, he sat with my son and reviewed the MRI images with him. He took my son in his lap, explaining to him the parts of the brain, how they work, and in his words, how beautiful that brain was, a huge tumor notwithstanding.

Every step of the way, Dr. Bhatia was with us, calming, assuring, supportive. On the day of the surgery, as he went over what to expect, my son looked at him, lifted his arm, and said, "Dr. Bhatia, while you're in there, can you take this splinter out of my arm? I've had it for a while." Without missing a beat, Dr. Bhatia took his marker and drew a circle around the splinter. We all kind of laughed it off and then left to wait through the grueling surgery that would take all day.

Hours later, when Dr. Bhatia came out to give us an update on the surgery, he asked us if we had any questions. My husband jokingly asked him if he had taken out the splinter. Smiling, Dr. Bhatia said, "That was the first thing I did." Sure enough, when we were able to finally see our son, he had a huge bandage around his head and a small one around his wrist.

It was a simple gesture that meant so much to my son and that most surgeons might have forgotten about and dismissed. But Dr. Bhatia seemed to always work from a position of humility and compassion, not ego and bravado. When the surgery was complete, my husband told Dr. Bhatia that thousands of people had been praying during the day throughout the procedure. Dr. Bhatia's simple response reflected his refined and unassuming personality: "I know. I felt it in my hands."

Dr. Bhatia was my son's friend through everything. With every MRI and every inpatient test, Dr. Bhatia was there, ready to make my son laugh, give him advice, and help us move away from those first fearful days and months. "Don't do drugs," he warned my son at our last visit. "I spent all this time fixing your brain, and then you're going to screw up my work?" And he always reminded us that he would personally write the recommendation letter to get my son into college. "I've seen your brain. You can do anything," he told my son.

To call Dr. Bhatia an angel might be clichéd, but I can't think of another term that sums up the beauty of this man's soul. I think of his delicate hands, his gentle voice, his laugh. I think of the power he held in that office, in that operating room, and in that hospital, and how we didn't even realize it because he never wielded it. All we knew was that he was saving our son, that he was fixing us. His medical recommendations for my son were given along with prescriptions for wine and a night out for me and my husband. He validated our concerns, assuaged our fears, and held our hands.

I never took a picture of my son with his favorite surgeon. I always wanted to wait until we were seeing him for the last time, not coming back for a follow-up, no longer worried about MRIs and symptoms. I didn't realize that this last visit would be the last time we would have that chance. Dr. Bhatia was a masterful, talented surgeon, a man who understood that removing a little boy's splinter was just as important as removing the tumor that was in his brain. His death leaves a void in the world, in the hospital, and in my heart. But I know, without a doubt, that the care he has given countless children and families, the benevolence and compassion that he bestowed on all of us, will remain with us. It will remind us how to act, how to be kind, and how to truly be a hero.

And I know I will miss him.

Wasn't Expecting This

It's been months since I've sat down to write. Months since we got news that we never wanted to hear, which I responded to with a carefully choreographed dance of denial and humor. When they put my son's latest MRI on the screen and started explaining what was there, I stopped the doctor to tell her that she had the wrong images. Those didn't belong to my son. It wasn't possible.

But willing it away was not a realistic approach, and so I sat there, stunned, as she discussed treatment options in the same way one would offer up candies or cake. I listened and nodded and ignored the roaring in my ears, the urge to run. I just sat there and watched as my life and my son's life changed completely and utterly once again.

My husband and I switched into research mode. I was back at the beginning, reading everything I could find, talking to anyone who had some insight, some connection to some random specialist who could direct us. I was a navigator, charting a course through waters I had never wanted to enter. I was pulling my son along for the ride, attaching him to me in a figurative flotation device, dragging him behind me as I launched through treacherous waves and uncharted territories. And even though I was so entrenched in it, I still did not believe it. I caught myself saying, "Okay, but this isn't, like, *real*," as I read off possible side effects and complications from treatments we were weighing.

It was much like that day three years ago when I sat dumbstruck by scans that could not be my son's. By news that could not possibly be for me.

It was a paradox that almost destroyed me. I had to move forward and focus, but at the same time, I was so desperate to erase the day I saw those images that I just tried to ignore the situation and pretend it never actually happened. I went back and forth from absolute calm to abject panic to crushing depression, then back to the warm blanket of denial.

My friends told me to write. It would be helpful. Maybe it would help me sort everything out. But there were no words to put on the page. Certainly nothing I wanted to see in print. Nothing I wanted to share with anyone. Because as I wrote this story, I would stop myself and say, "No. This isn't real. This isn't true," like a child closing her eyes and covering her ears, believing it would make everything go away.

Crises explode with seeming chaos, but pain has a precise trajectory when it's gunning for your child. It is a targeted attack on the soul, reverberating to your heart and refocusing every ounce of your being into survival mode. The responses of denial, of outrage, and even of humor, are just different Band-Aids for the same wound. A wound that can only be fixed with hope, with love, with faith, with friends, and agonizingly, with time.

Months later, I'm swimming more smoothly out on that menacing sea. There are still so many unknowns. So many days when I wish I could find that castle of denial again and take up residence inside it. But now, I don't have that luxury. I can look at this situation, recognize it for what it is, and focus on moving through it. And my family will move through it. We already are.

I hadn't written since the day I sat in front of the screen looking at those new MRI images. It was too huge. Too all consuming. It dwarfed my stupid ideas and silly blogs. But here it is, here I am: raw, unedited, as I see it and feel it. I never expected to be here. I never expected to write about this again. I never expected to be blindsided like that. I never expected to be floundering on that sinister ocean, trying to keep myself and my family afloat.

I never expected any of this.

But now, I no longer have any expectations.

For now, it's about getting back into the ring, one foot in front of the other. For now, it's just about moving forward.

"Oh. Okay. So We're Good?"

There is plenty of advice out there when it comes to comforting the weary. Things not to say and things to say. How to offer help. How to listen. How to be compassionate. The advice doesn't really matter, because having been on both sides of the comforter/comfortee scenario, I know that it's pretty hard not to screw it up anyway. Maybe it's because we're all so different, and so one person's words of comfort are another person's proverbial fingernails scratching on the blackboard. It's hard to gauge.

I don't claim to be an expert on offering support, but lately, the overly positive "tell me good news" responses are high on my list of things not to do. I'm thinking that maybe it's because no one wants to be a downer. If your friend is in a difficult place, the knee-jerk reaction is to put a positive spin on things. It's the rah-rah-rah of the cancer-ward orderly. The pink-clad cheerleader at the 5K. The smiling, pastel-lipsticked neighbor who brings over the casserole. And there is a place for bringing happiness and joy to serious situations. Even an unsolicited casserole. I'm not knocking that.

But within the quest to comfort and help, the desire for positivity often becomes an unintentional dismissal of the severity of a situation. No one genuinely wants to add pain to someone else's difficulty, and so the fallback, the easiest response, is to try to reframe the pain into something manageable. Try to find the silver lining hovering around the sick and miserable rain cloud. What's left is the default response of "Oh. Okay. So that's good."

There are various forms of it. When I was first leaving town with my youngest son to meet with doctors out of state and decide on treatment options for his recurrent brain tumor, my friend told me that she was "looking forward to hearing good news." I looked at her and, in a burst of frustration and misplaced anger, blurted that there won't be any good news. I was looking at treatment plans, not miracles. The only news I was going to be bringing back was just levels of bad. Would we choose the option that destroyed his liver or his kidneys? Would we risk hearing loss or vision problems? We would not come home with good news , and her glossy, well-meaning sentiment left me hollow. It only highlighted the difference between the pre–brain tumor world I used to live in and the one where I currently reside. She didn't have a clue. There was no way she could.

At every corner, friends and relatives have been quick to say "Oh. Okay. So that's good" to small points of whatever new development I share. But none of it is good. It is unfathomable. It is terrible. It is terrifying. And the more positivity that is thrown at me, the more I want to scream.

I've stopped sharing information, or rather, I do so selectively. It isn't that I am wallowing in darkness and brooding over my personal pain. It's that my reality is difficult, and I need to address it pragmatically. Without platitudes and rainbows. My rejection of their positivity isn't an embrace of negativity and cynicism. Rather, it is the understanding that their misplaced encouragement has little to do with my current reality. As such, their words make that reality seem like a triviality they can dismiss with a sweeping assessment of, "Okay. So we're good." The world wants to hear the good stuff. They want to make everything better with a casserole and some cheerleaders. They want the happy ending, and I am still far from that chapter.

Because it doesn't just end with those beginning days either. Only someone who has been on the illness side of the coin knows that being in the clear takes years. That our lives have been permanently changed. That even as we smile for the family pictures, nothing is ever the same. And so people's desire to put the experience into a shiny box, clap a hand on my shoulder, and say, "Oh. Okay. So, we're good?"—as if my family can return to business as usual—is unrealistic and virtually impossible.

And yet, there it is, everywhere.

I think I've come a long way since that moment when I yelled at my friend. After all, I know that the positive vibes and good wishes are coming from a place of love and caring. I also recognize that I'm no longer on the same planet as some of my closest friends. Not by any fault of their own, but because there is no common ground anymore when I'm in hospitals and office buildings they will thankfully, I hope, never have to visit with their child.

I don't know how to comfort the bereaved or the sick or the weary, even though I've been on that side numerous times. There is no magic formula, regardless of what that article taped to your fridge says. But if there is one constant, I think it is the need to recognize struggle. The need to accept someone's painful reality. The need to be present during hard times, sometimes in silence, and oftentimes without a casserole.

Bringing light to darkness doesn't always mean pointing out the good. It means standing by your friend as she finds it herself. And being there to celebrate those moments when she offers up, on her own, "Okay. I'm good."

On Parties and CT Scans

It's been four years to the day since I sat with my husband and our parents, waiting for our youngest son to come out of surgery for a brain tumor. It was a very long day, a grueling surgery, and the launching point for a new life we never knew was coming. I usually post my blog entry from two years ago when I reflect on what this anniversary means, but this year I'm writing from a different place.

I mean that literally.

This year, as the anniversary of that surgery popped onto my newsfeed like a happy cheerleader ("We thought you'd like to look back on these memories today, Adina!"), I was in the emergency room with that same child. I was waiting for him to return from a CT scan, hoping that the pain he was in was just some random incident and not further progression of this recurrent disease that has shadowed most of our days for four years.

It was an ironic moment. The doctors wheeled him out of our cheerfully decorated little ER room and, smiling, said they'd be right back, that they were sure he'd be fine. It took me back to when my husband and I were handed a similar narrative that never played out the way it was supposed to. Back then, I thought we were dealing with a sprint—a short moment that would end with a happily ever after and a quick blog post about blessings and family. But I'm a bit jaded now, and so their words of comfort filled me with a sense of dread instead of relief.

I glanced at my phone and watched as the date changed from May 6 to May 7, and I realized that it's four years later and I'm waiting in a hospital. Again.

Once we knew we were going to the ER, I packed a quick bag, taking my laptop and chargers, a fuzzy blanket, and changes of clothes for everyone. It was easy to pack, having done it numerous times in the past. You know you've reached a bizarre moment in your life when you can walk through an emergency room and request one bay that you know is "better" than another.

"Can we get the Panther room? We like that one."

So I sat there with my laptop, working on—of all things— Bar Mitzvah invitations for the kid in the CT scanner. My husband sat next to me, saw what I was doing, and after an awkward moment of silence, both of us just started laughing. It was probably a combination of stress and scanxiety. It was the ridiculousness that we are still dealing with hospitals and doctors, and the realization that we have no idea what the next five minutes will bring, much less the next few years. The absurdity of planning a celebration while waiting for what could be bad news.

I wax poetic about medicine these days. Having moved from the world of the twenty-four-hour virus, to the ten-day course of antibiotics, to the unending and nebulous realm of brain tumors and treatments, I recently made peace with what will be a long-term situation. Gone are the days where we plan for the summer "when everything is finished" or for the party that will be a "celebration of everything turning out great!" Our reality shifted somewhere along the line, putting us in a place where we can wait for CT results while planning a party that we are both hesitant to put on. We can't wait for the perfect summer, the perfect date, the perfect moment when these past four years will be a blip on the screen. The past four years have *become* the screen, and we get that it is our responsibility to meld it into our reality instead of bemoaning its presence. It is part of what they keep telling us is our new normal, an aspect of life that demands we still live despite the ever-present shadows.

It's why, four years after that gun went off, I sit in an emergency room at 1:00 a.m. and fix invitation designs and think about centerpieces at the same time my son is returning from a scan, and pain medication and drugs to help him sleep are being pushed into his IV. It's what we have to do. It's what we always do.

Four years out, and it's taken me this long to understand the difference between a marathon and a sprint.

Happy anniversary.

Happiness and Stingrays

I learned a powerful lesson about happiness from my thirteen-year-old son.

We were driving home from a doctor's appointment, and out of nowhere he said, "I feel bad for stingrays."

He had once seen stingrays at our local science museum, and so I figured he was talking about how terrible it is that the stingrays are captives—unable to swim in the ocean or get away from the little kids that reach their hands into the display to try to grab at them.

But he had a different take.

"I feel bad for the stingrays. They're always smiling, but only because they have to. They're probably sad and no one even knows."

Do a quick Google search of stingrays and you'll see what he means. They have these goofy grins that make them look like they're gently smiling at the world, happily gliding through the water. Their faces are frozen in place like Wybie in *Coraline*. They look like that all the time, but it isn't a "real" smile. After all, the stingray that killed Steve Irwin was also "smiling."

My son's words were poetic and tragic, providing insight into his own life and into the world around him. So many people we encounter—who smile and smile—do so not because they are truly happy but because they have no choice. They put their smile out there for everyone to see, to keep people at bay, to avoid dealing with the inquisitive minds or the nagging questions. It's so much easier to paint on the smile and let the world assume that everything is good. Everything is fine.

Maybe the lesson of the stingrays is to keep smiling regardless of your circumstances. Even if you're trapped in a museum, getting grabbed at by screeching toddlers and their parents. Even if you're confined and unable to swim out to your ocean. It's the smile of inner strength and fortitude.

Or maybe the stingray offers a complex lesson about our own interpersonal relationships, the reminder that we shouldn't take the outward smiles for granted and make assumptions. Everyone carries pain. Some are just better at hiding it. Some are better at keeping the grin plastered on forever, swimming in the stifling environment of the man-made tide pool, burying the anguish behind sad eyes so that no one notices. Not all who smile are happy.

More than likely, it's both those lessons.

I have told my children that it is important to not let pain or tragedy define who they are. To not let it become their identity. And so that means they must endeavor, even in times of difficulty, to find something to smile about, things to celebrate, or they will have no choice but to stay in bed, eat chocolate, and succumb to the darkness that is everywhere. It's a philosophy that is easy to preach but difficult to practice, and they sometimes get angry when I try to spin things to the positive. I know there are times I also want to wallow in the bad and lash out at positivity and silver linings.

And I often do. Which is why the second lesson is so important as well. Having been touched by pain, it is also our job to look beyond the smiles. To recognize that all who smile are carrying burdens we know nothing about. To be there for others, to open the door, to let them know "It's okay, you don't have to smile all the time. I know what it's like."

Recently, my son had a bad reaction to anesthesia from an MRI and wound up damaging his eye. He was in pain and couldn't see for two days. His eyes were bandaged *Birdbox* style, and I joked with him that we would reenact scenes from that movie until his eyes were better. He asked me to take a picture so he could see what he looked like, and I did, thinking it would be a picture for him alone. But looking at it now, it's remarkable. He was in a lot of pain and was scared, but you wouldn't know it. He was *smiling*.

It was a smile of strength. It was the smile of the stingray.

Dueling with God

Next week is Rosh Hashanah, the beginning of the holiest days in the Jewish calendar. It's when we pray for a good and sweet year and ask God to inscribe us in the Book of Life.

Lately, it seems like my interactions with God have been more adversarial than comforting. We meet daily for an Old West–style shootout. Sometimes at 1:00 a.m., sometimes at 5:00 a.m., sometimes at midday. Just me and Him. No red strings or lucky eye charms. The God I meet is not a Cracker Jack kind of being. No superstitions or silly wand-waving. It is just us.

There's only one bullet in the chamber each day. And we spin it blindly, face off, and take aim.

I know that every day I might get hit with the bullet. I know that each day I am sitting at the end of our pseudo–Russian roulette, and sometimes it's a blank. But the gun is always there.

Sometimes it is pointed at someone else. When I happen upon another duel on my figurative street, I become an interloper to someone else's pain. I jump in front of the gun and yell, "No! Not her. Not him. Not that family." I cry and plead and beg for the gun to be lowered, for the barrel to be empty, for it to be leveled at me instead. Though when I sense it might be, I quickly fall back to my default: "No. Not me. Not my child. Not my family."

So when we face off again in our daily duel, I carry the guilt of having survived the last few rounds when I know others have not, and I tempt Him again to take His best shot. I wonder if this is the day the bullet is in the chamber, or if it will just be the click of the hammer and I can walk away unscathed.

There are others, I know. People who never realize there is a daily duel. People who come to the street dancing and singing and don't notice the revolver, the slowly turning barrel, the click of the hammer on an empty chamber. I envy them sometimes. The people who lament the skinned knees. The people who plead with God to get their children into college. Never realizing what they are dodging as they grieve the inconsequential.

But lately, I fear that duel. Not because of the bullet that might find its way to my life from His side, but because of the gun in my hand. The times that I sometimes want to say, "That's it! I'm done! This makes no sense!" The moments when I would find so much more sense in science and technology and randomness than in a daily duel with a God who doesn't always seem to listen to my pleas.

And so we duel. Day after day. On my runs in the morning and late at night in my bedroom. The hours tick by, and I wait for Him to show up so I can shake my fist, or lower my head resignedly, or maybe, fire my own gun back.

It has taken some time, but I've made a tacit peace with the duel. I recognize that for some reason, God is dragging me onto that street, and despite my pleas and cries to avoid the duel, He insists on it. Insists on placing that gun in my hands, insists on spinning the chamber. Insists on tempting me to draw and shoot. And so maybe my pleas about the bullet are really about the duel itself and just wanting a simple relationship with God again. Maybe it's about wishing I could go back to dancing in that same street, oblivious and blind to the constant threats, content with ignorance and naïveté.

For the last few years, my daily duel with God has grown more intense. I never shoot back, though the gun has always been in my hand. I never pull the trigger. Because as easy as it would be to do, to take aim and try to end the constant duel once and for all, I know I need that daily meeting. I know I need to have someone to plead with, to pray to, to ask things of. My duel with God, then, is in some small way an affirmation of my faith.

This Rosh Hashanah, I'm not dueling with God. We'll meet, I'm sure, in the center of the street, shake hands, and look over our weapons. We'll spin our barrels and walk back to our corners, setting up for the coming year of struggles. We'll face off numerous times this coming year, but after all this time, I finally recognize that between our duels, there are moments of beauty and love. My duel with God might frame our relationship, but it also keeps it intact. It keeps Him present in a complex, deep, and sometimes frustrating way, as a partner in both pain and joy.

He knows me well. He also knows that regardless of the bullet's trajectory, I have every intention of meeting Him every day, and remaining standing.

It's been years of dueling. I'm still here on that street. And more importantly, so is He.

One Photo

With everyone holed up in their homes trying to keep their families safe during the pandemic lockdowns, I've been challenged on a nearly constant basis. These aren't the challenges you would think. I'm talking about the photo challenges, the book challenges, the recipe challenges. It seems like everyone is so desperate for entertainment that everything is suddenly a challenge.

"I've been challenged to post the titles of ten novels."

"I've been challenged to post pictures of motherhood."

"I've been challenged to post my favorite dinners."

I kind of laugh at them because the nasty, sarcastic part of me wants to respond with, "Honey, if that's your challenge, we should talk."

But not wanting to be that person, and recognizing that it's all in good fun, I just roll my eyes and scroll past. Engaging in social media these days sometimes requires more emotional effort than I'm willing to invest, and so I like the challenges I'm tagged in and just move on without joining the flurry of photo-posting and social gushing.

Today is a bit harder.

I got a message to join the photo challenge. "Post one picture every day for ten days that has meaning to you. Don't comment. Just post it. And challenge someone else every day." Normally, I would do what I always do: like, smiley face, move on. But today, I'm thinking about one picture. One photo that has more meaning to me than any other. And so this innocuous, meaningless challenge, on today of all days, sent me off to the races.

Every year, for the past five years, there has been only one photo I think of on this day, May 7. It isn't the one you would think. It's not a picture of my son post-surgery in the hospital, or a picture of us in the waiting room on that long day. The picture I always think of is this one:

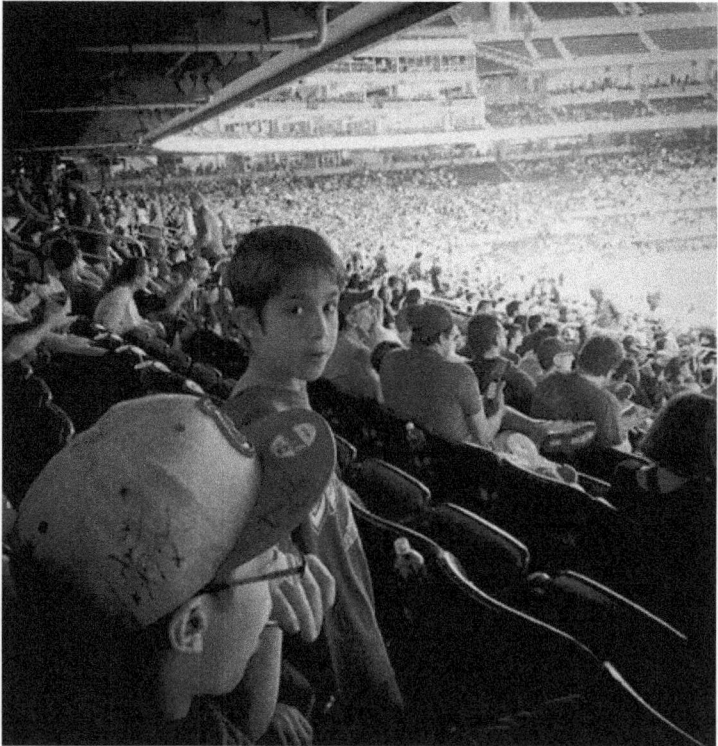

This is at a Marlins game in April 2015. Twenty-four hours after this picture was taken, I was in the ER with my son, finding out he had a brain tumor. To me, this picture is the ultimate "before" shot. I was at the game with all my kids. Everyone was somewhat miserable because it was so hot, and the game was so slow. I had forced them all to go, and I knew they were all humoring me. I took this picture on a whim, not realizing how much our lives would change within one day and how this one picture would reflect an entire world that I would leave behind twenty-four hours later. The picture is different for me than for anyone else who might look at it. I could post it on that stupid photo challenge and no one would know why I chose it. "Cute pic!" someone might say, not realizing that in the realm of challenges, this photo knocks almost all others out of the *actual* ballpark.

I'd like to think that I could look at this one photo and scroll on the way I do with these inane challenges and posts. But five years later, I'm having a tough time getting through this day, more so than in years before. Maybe it's because five years ago, the plan seemed optimistic, and now I've come to a place of uncomfortable peace with the uncertainty that fills every day and probably will fill every day for the next five years. And maybe the next five years after that.

Or maybe it's that the stress of keeping my family safe has finally reached a tipping point, today of all days, where the patience I've been practicing is no longer at my fingertips. That when I see photo challenges and mournful posts about the difficulties of lockdown, I scroll past, but that very real desire to lash out at the poster with "You want a challenge?!" has moved closer to the surface. While the world cries about toilet paper and yeast and sacrificing the "immunoscrewed," it takes every ounce of strength to not post the photo of my son's chemotherapy drugs—the one thing *we* have been hoarding.

I also know I'm unreasonable. I know everyone is having a hard time. I know stocks are crashing, unemployment is high, people are scared. I know this is a bad time to argue the semantics of "challenge," but today, even amid worldwide chaos, I'm back to five years ago, looking at a picture that reminds me of how life changes on a dime.

It's five years later. It's two years since we had to step back into the ring. It's fifteen months since we started treatment, and we're hoping for the best. So many photos have been taken between that one at the stadium and the one from dinner last night, each one telling the story in moments and pieces and different anniversaries.

Maybe I'm being hard on the photo challenge. Maybe the challenge isn't in finding the photos, it's in refraining from comment and engaging in reflection. Simply looking at it and saying, with no backstory or pretense, "This is my photo. This is my life. This is my challenge."

Happy anniversary.

Chesed Bitches

che·sed

/'KHesəd/

noun JUDAISM

1. the attribute of grace, benevolence, or compassion, especially (in Kabbalism) as one of the sephiroth.

I've had it with the Chesed Bitches. The ones who show up at the door, lasagna pans in hand, all smiles and cheerfulness, to help the bereaved and the sick. They are the first to sign up on the meal trains, the first to sponsor an ill child. They are the designated mourners and the people perpetually tracking the pulses of the downtrodden and the unfortunate.

I know. I sound ungrateful. But I'm not. Because there's a difference between "true" chesed and what my daughter and I lovingly refer to as the Chesed Bitches.

True chesed is making a meal for someone in need, helping where needed, taking care of things that fall to the side when someone is thrown into crisis. Some people, though, do those things not for the families they are supposedly helping but for their own sense of self-worth. They are the people who make meals when no one asked because "I know you really want this, and anyway, you can freeze it for later." They post their good deeds on social media with #BlessedToHelp or #HelpingTheSick to announce to everyone what they are doing. They want the world to know that they started the prayer group, that they launched the Go Fund Me, that they deserve a chesed trophy or a sparkling medal. Like a little award at assembly time in high school.

I've seen them in full force. Having your family hit by cancer twice will bring them out in droves. They arrived in the form of unsolicited advice and Google searches they clearly didn't imagine we'd thought of. They arrived with Facebook posts that bordered on abusive, all under the guise of "I'm just trying to help." My friend had to rent a second freezer to store the unsolicited food trays people brought over to "make things easier." Another friend begged people to take the lunch a well-meaning person had brought to her shiva house when it was already bursting with meals and frozen dishes. The food was not a help—it was just another thing to worry about.

Chesed—the act of helping someone in need—is first and foremost an act of giving to the person or family. The narcissistic twist that chesed has been getting, fueled by social media and the need to post everything these days, has changed the playing field. I think it's important to recognize the difference between acting for others and acting for one's own personal sense of fulfillment. No matter how well-meaning the intention, it is imperative to keep the object of the chesed in mind. You might be able to make a mean lasagna, but if someone says "Please don't," you need to respect that.

When my son came out of surgery, we asked people not to come to the hospital. I received a text when I was in the ICU that said, "I know you said you didn't want visitors, but I knew you really did. So I'm here. Can you tell the doctors to let me in?" I was mildly horrified and couldn't believe that she hadn't listened when I said, "Please no visitors."

Sigh.

Chesed Bitches.

As I said before, I know I sound ungrateful. But really, it's not ingratitude. I am grateful to the people who reached out and really helped us. But it's difficult to find yourself in a position to require help. There were people who helped with a full heart and no ulterior motives, and there were a lot of them. They were the ones who truly saved us during times of crisis. But in between the genuine good, there is always the person who is working for reasons that have nothing to do with pain or tragedy.

I'm not someone's pet project to make themselves feel better. And if that's what's motivating you, then that's not chesed, bitch.

Not Today

I was late to the *Game of Thrones* party. When everyone was posting their reactions to each episode and season, I was ignoring it all, not investing in the excitement. So when I decided to binge all eight seasons in one summer, it was a somewhat lonely experience. I finally understood the hype and wanted to talk to people about each episode, but they had all moved on. I was alone.

What I found so compelling about *Game of Thrones* wasn't just the plot twists and the character arcs. It was the real-life comparisons I saw everywhere. I saw it played out in politics, in relationships, in everyday experiences. *Game of Thrones* was a larger metaphor constantly unfolding around me. It became a subtle teacher, giving me a guide for how to behave and interact and play the figurative "game of thrones" we all face daily.

I was recently reminded of this on a particularly grueling medical trip with my youngest son. As a parent, once you've crossed the threshold from childhood illnesses to tumor treatments, it's easy to catastrophize any symptoms and weird behaviors that your child exhibits. On this trip, we had a lot of that. One situation almost caused an emergency landing on our flight. It was a trip fraught with unexplained crisis after crisis, and everything was pointing in a bad direction. I thought I would lose my mind. Knowing that I was probably a poor judge of my own sanity and worried that maybe I was imagining things, I reached out to my friend and asked him if he thought I was going crazy.

His answer went back to *Game of Thrones*. Specifically, to one line.

"Remember Arya Stark," he said, reminding me of the character who watched her family get murdered one by one and exacted revenge through six seasons of the show. "You're living in a world beyond imagining. Like Arya, the threats are existential. She responded to them by becoming a badass assassin and learning to fight in the dark. That's what you have to do." And then he reminded me of the line Arya learned from the first person who taught her how to fight:

"What do we say to the god of death? Not today."

Way back when I was finding out I had breast cancer, people would tell me to "be strong," as if I actually had anything to do with the fight. Things were happening *to* me—I was getting surgery. I was given drugs. I was having tests. The only battle I really had was with post-cancer depression and the well-meaning toxic positivity that tended to blow up my phone on bad days. More often than not, I felt like a victim, not a fighter, regardless of what all the movie lines said. I gave in to that passiveness with the mantra of "Day by day." I just had to get through the four hours for another Percocet. Get through the six hours for more Dilaudid. Get through the day. Get through the next day. And that was how it went.

Arya's "Not today," on the other hand, is active. It implies fighting and strength. It is a call not only in direct defiance to the god of death, but to the gods of chaos and crisis. There is nothing passive about it. It reminds you to dig deep, to raise your sword and threaten the darkness that seeks to overwhelm you. It reminds you to get back into the ring instead of lying down or losing yourself within it.

The difference between "Day by day" and "Not today" is the difference between passivity and action. "Day by day" forces you to watch and wait until the danger passes. Let it wash over you. Accept it. There certainly is a time and a place for that advice. It's the same advice I received about labor: breathe into the pain, wait for the contraction to end, get your breath, do it again.

When I was watching my kid going through crisis, my knee-jerk mom reaction was to give him the same mantra. Day by day. Test by test. Pill by pill. But this time around, he wasn't buying it. This time, like me, he needed a sword. He needed to face off with the god of death. He needed to look the pain in the eye and resolutely say, no matter how large the fear and the unknown, "Not today."

It may have taken me longer to get to *Game of Thrones* than most people, but because the experience is still so fresh, my friend's reminder of Arya battling in darkness resonated so well. But you don't need to be familiar with the storyline to recognize the difference between the approaches. When faced with pain, with the unknown, with visions of worst-case scenarios—when you're fighting in darkness—there is really only one way to respond.

Only one thing we say to that.

Not today.

Not today.

Not today.

Scanxiety

"So how'd it go?"

"**The MRI is** (*supposed to be only an hour and a half but he was in there for two and a half hours while I paced outside, vacillating between panic and despair and internal reprimands of thinking positive, especially since we had traveled to get this scan on the best machine, and the doctors are not expecting anything dramatic since he hasn't had any symptoms recently, but of course that means nothing because he didn't have any symptoms the first time either and we know how that worked out, plus I have noticed that he's been tired more often lately and he totally can't concentrate even though he is doing well in school, but that doesn't mean anything either because even if he's getting straight A's, they keep reminding us that it's probably only a matter of time before he will need more treatment, and he's already so sick of medication and doctors and missing school and putting on MRI scrubs and those horrible socks that they try to make cheerful and cute with the bear paws, but c'mon, he's fourteen and that doesn't work anymore, like the anesthesia that is supposed to smell like strawberries but just smells like those dangling tree-shaped air*

185

fresheners, and even though it knocks him out, it can't taste good for those few seconds, especially since it probably reminds him of the Uber we were just in to get here at this ungodly hour where I hang out in freezing rooms with bad coffee and worse lighting, ignoring text messages and scrolling though TikTok for the hours that he's in there so I don't have to think about the hours he's been in there because there was probably a complication, like his breathing stopped or he had a seizure or he finally got a reaction to the gadolinium, and about how awful it is that I can just call up that word so easily, along with the brand names of chemo drugs and inhibitor drugs and all their side effects, and that I can read through new advances in cancer research and brain tumors as casually as BuzzFeed articles that make no difference for the here and now in the MRI waiting area where I fill out the forms for copies of the CD so that when I'm home, I can pop it in my ancient computer that I keep only because it still has a CD player that lets me scour the images for hours, pretending I know what I'm looking at and seeing cancer everywhere because even before I refreshed MyChart for the millionth time that day, knowing that the report would not have been uploaded so quickly, I convinced myself that we are getting bad news and know that even if we aren't, we will still be back in this same place again and again with the dreary socks and the all-too-bright rooms and the warmed-up blankets that don't keep him cozy past the first few minutes and my smile that I've kept plastered on my face for the past two weeks up until this point in a futile attempt to 'think positive,' even though I know he sees through it and thankfully never calls me on it, with the tacit reminder that rears its head each time we are here that maybe we are on borrowed time, and all we can hope is that one day our lives will once again be) **stable**."

"Amazing! You must be so happy!"

Evil Decrees

One of the most famous prayers in the Rosh Hashanah and Yom Kippur service is the prayer of "Unesaneh Tokef." The prayer describes exactly what God writes on Rosh Hashana, and what He seals on Yom Kippur. The words provide a menu of ways to die—from stoning to drowning, from plague to starvation—and a description of other negative events that may befall you. Your fate for the year is pretty much written in the books during these high holy days.

The final line of the prayer, though, reminds us that nothing is set in stone: "Repentance, Prayer, and Charity can avert the evil decree." It's a simple three-step-process for making sure we are written in the Book of Life, and that whatever decree was meant for us can be averted through our good deeds.

At least, I *used* to think that was what the prayer was about.

Maybe it was a bit of confirmation bias and the years of Yeshiva Day School that taught me what the final line said. But this year, I actually read it carefully and noticed that the last line of the prayer does not say anything of the sort. Translated exactly, the final line reads: "Repentance, Prayer, and Charity can avert the evil of the decree." We're not averting the decree itself, just the evilness of it.

It's a subtle difference that changes the entire meaning. Looking back into the text at the list of ways to die, the new reading seems to imply that there is no way to escape the decrees of death and destruction. But it isn't as fatalistic as it sounds. The text doesn't say, "*You* might drown. *You* might die by plague." It says that God decides *who* that will happen to, me and you being two of those possibilities. The poem is simply stating an obvious idea. Death, pain, suffering—these are things we are all going to experience this year. We can't escape it. If it is not us, it will be someone we know. Something we will witness.

The last line, then, the one about repentance, prayer, and charity, is not a line giving us a recipe to make it all go away. Bad things will always exist in this world. Instead, it's giving us tools to cope with the evil that we may experience. It's telling us that to get rid of the evil of the decree, we need to do three things: look inward to ourselves, look up to God, and give back to our community. By looking inward, I can examine what this experience has done to me, what I can get out of it. How I can change from it. By looking up to God, I have someone to rail at, to duel with, to question. And by giving to my community, I can turn my experience into a positive. I can create a legacy. I can turn tragedy into positive action.

Rosh Hashanah and Yom Kippur are days that focus on those relationships. It's a communal meditation on ourselves, God, and our friends. What the poet is telling us in this universal prayer is that we are not going to escape trauma and pain. We can't stop that from happening. But those experiences do not have to destroy us, our relationships, and our connections.

I have seen destruction happen to people I love who have experienced tragedy and pain. I have also been on the other side, the receiver of evil decrees, and I have struggled to make sense of hardships when there is no answer for suffering.

It isn't easy.

The prayer for the new year is not a message of false hope, of a year without pain, but rather a guide for enduring that weariness, a reminder of the hackneyed expression that while pain is inevitable, suffering is a choice. These inescapable, painful decrees can lose their destructive, evil nature and instead become catalysts for change and growth, if we heed the words of the poet: look inward, reach upward, branch outward.

On Anniversaries

As a kid, the only anniversary in my life belonged to my parents. I only understood the concept in terms of weddings. Fast forward a few years, and I celebrated the inane anniversaries of high-school romances: anniversary of a first date, anniversary of a first ice cream, anniversaries of other firsts that I thought would signify my forever romance or turn into, maybe, the celebration of a wedding.

Back then, anniversaries were always celebrations of happiness, recalling a day or moment when life changed for the better. Those still exist, but somewhere in the past few years, the more pervasive anniversaries of sad days moved into my life. It's possible it's just a consequence of growing older, the rosy-hued days of youth giving way to the jaded and complex days of adulthood. But recently, I started rethinking the days that we give meaning to, the days that we pause to remember some event—both good and bad.

I used to pause on the anniversary of my mastectomy. It's coming up soon, and so is the necessary contemplation that goes along with it. In cancer groups, people discuss celebrating their "Cancerversaries," marking the day they were diagnosed with some gallows-humor fanfare. Like piping "Congratulations on Not Dying!" in pink frosting on chocolate cakes, or celebrating "Rebirthdays" on the day they received lifesaving stem cells. It's a staple for some, but triggering for others who believe that reminders of the past should maybe just stay in the past.

I'm on the fence in the debate. Sometimes I bristle at it. Other times I embrace it. Regardless, when certain dates creep up in the calendar, I find myself mentally gearing up for it like a birthday—knowing it's there, year after year, the same mix of bitter and sweet.

On the first anniversary of my son's diagnosis, I locked the doors and wouldn't let anyone out of the house, thinking that by keeping everyone home, nothing could happen. That we would get past the day unscathed. And even though I knew that particular day was no different from the day before except in the number on the calendar, keeping everyone in one place gave me a childish sense of control. If we escape the day, we will survive the year. I won't be surprised again. Won't be caught off-guard. That day, as long as I remember it, will be a safe day.

I can't keep my family locked up every year, and I can't sit here and wait with bated breath for catastrophe to strike. Balancing the acknowledgment of an anniversary without emotionally returning to those moments takes time. Marking the day isn't choosing to stay in that past; rather, it is an affirmation of the future. The years that tick down after an "anniversary" are proof of the constancy of life and happiness in the face of difficult days and struggles.

We celebrate the anniversary of a wedding, pause and reflect on the anniversary of a tragedy, and ultimately contemplate all the anniversaries that make up the fabric of a life lived and experienced.

Today is an anniversary I remember each year, holding it for a few moments as a reminder of where I was and where I am now. It's taken a while to realize that though the day looms heavy on the calendar, giving myself space to recognize it does not give it power, does not send me into hiding in my home.

All our days are anniversaries of something. Sometimes you don't realize the implications of a day's events. Other times, those events explode in your face, leaving a day that is forever scarred, leaving you with an anniversary you would never wish for.

The anniversaries in my life are a mix of celebrations and contemplations that battle each other for prominence. I count down toward those days on the calendar in both expectation and apprehension. They are the scaffolding that make up the cataclysmic moments in life—both good and bad—that demand some type of meditation.

This is my meditation. This is my anniversary.

Happy anniversary.

A Thank-You Letter to My Insurance Company upon Denying the Claim for My Kid's Medication for the Fourth Time

Dear Favorite Insurance Company,

Thank you so much for denying the claim for the recommended medication for our child! We never knew how creative we could get with brain tumor cures until you went against three doctors and a surgeon to base your final decision on the vast medical knowledge of Tom in Accounting. In these days of misinformation and blind trust in science, it is good to know that our health-care team explores alternative sources of information and allows us access to tried-and-true techniques like "bloodletting" and "keeping a positive attitude." We are so lucky to be on your plan!

We know we owe you some money, but fear not. Even with the impending foreclosure and upcoming bankruptcy, and even though we are buying Ativan for cash from the alley behind the drugstore, we have designated *you* as the first group to get payments from our GoFundMe! Because what could be more important than having our team of insurance agents cheer us along and drag out treatment as long as possible so we can experience the sheer exhilaration of watching our deductible reset on January 1? Seriously, we cannot even express how excited we are for that day. Most people watch the countdown to the New Year from Times Square, but lucky us, we do it from your user-friendly dashboard. You should definitely consider adding a confetti effect at midnight to sweeten the moment. That would be adorable.

Speaking of suggestions, do not—and I mean do NOT—change that glorious hold music! Having listened to it for upward of five hundred hours, I think I am in the position to tell you that you need to take it on the road. Why deny the world the beauty of a sharply volume-shifting, repetitive tune that evokes the wonder of being trapped in an underwater cavern without oxygen? And with my heart rate rising with each passing minute, it's like I'm getting a workout while I wait for my claims denials. So clever!

Without you, we would probably be spending our money on trivialities like filling our car with gas, buying canned beans, or saving our son from unnecessary pain, and so we thank you for keeping us grounded and focused on the important things. Like learning how to pole dance at a local club to score some sample-size Zofran tabs from the doctors who show up in the front row. Can't even tell you how exciting it is to feel that smooth, child-resistant plastic bottle tucked into my bikini strap instead of cash! And no copay!

Even without the medication that you keep denying us, we realize that as health-care providers, you have our best interests at heart. And if that means making sure we are in prime condition to be contestants on *Survivor*, well then, all we can say once again is thank you.

Your bestie,
Adina

Not My God, Not My Religion

Our family recently had a bit of a health scare.

Don't worry, everything is fine. We are all fine. There's nothing to report or discuss.

But about a month and a half ago, things weren't so fine. We were worried that maybe we would have to write a post that wasn't so positive. That maybe our good run was over. That we were back at the beginning again.

In some ways, we were. We were waiting for test results for scans ordered by my oncologist. Waiting to find out if I would have to take a leave of absence from work. Waiting to see if life was going to turn around and try to kick us down the way it has in the past.

Whenever there is some sort of chaos or crisis in our lives, well-meaning friends are quick to come out of the woodwork and remind us of some things we should do. Pray. Say psalms. Give charity. And the all-important, always ready, always doable: check your mezuzahs.

We've checked them a bunch of times since moving into our new home. Removing them from the doorposts, bringing them to a rabbi who either tells us they're fine or finds some letter scratched out, some phrase that is missing. And so we replace these doorway sentinels, hoping that repairing the letters will fix whatever ailments are plaguing us.

But not this time.

This time, when things started going south, we didn't share the grim news with anyone. I had called my husband from the hospital with news that my PET scan had lit up where it wasn't supposed to and we needed to follow up with more tests. Things would go one of two ways—either everything was fine, or everything was not fine. There was no in between. Before he responded, I warned him: "If you take one mezuzah down from any doorpost, I'm divorcing you."

I could not take down those mezuzahs again. Could not believe that a letter scratched out had cursed us in some way. I could not buy into it anymore—that God would choose to punish us over something so small. That if only we had checked them earlier, maybe my son would not have had a brain tumor. Maybe I wouldn't have had breast cancer. Maybe.

I decided right then that I couldn't believe in that God of superstition and amulets and magical talismans. That isn't my religion. That isn't my God.

My friend Rachel said it best. When I told her a bit of what was happening and my changing feelings about the protection those mezuzahs were supposed to give, she agreed. Not everything has a clear reason. We don't know why bad things happen. And more importantly, she explained, "The God I believe in is crying with me. He's sad too. And He certainly isn't blaming me."

The theological crisis that arises from tragedy and pain is an old story. I'm not one to pontificate on where God was when I was going through difficult times. In fact, I didn't really have much time to think about where He was, other than to pray that He would somehow come through. But while I can question why things happened the way they did, why we keep finding new battles, and why we can't seem to close the metaphorical door of our situation, I can't buy into the simple notion that "if only we had checked the mezuzahs" or "if only we had prayed harder" or—and this was real—"if only I would have worn longer skirts," then none of this would have happened.

It's easy to find something to pinpoint as the cause of our suffering. It's a natural desire. Having no answers doesn't work in our data-driven, logical, grounded minds. How simple is it to point to external factors—the mezuzahs on the doors, the quality of our prayers, the length of our skirts—so we can turn around and say, "Aha! That's why this happened! Fix it, and all your troubles will go away!"

That isn't the God I believe in. My God is much more complex. Much deeper. And certainly not so petty as to make us suffer for lack of a letter on a piece of parchment nailed to our doors. I would much rather file my troubles in a folder that's labeled "I Don't Understand" than point to a talisman and blame it on that. I don't mind having a God that I sometimes don't understand. A God that I sometimes question. A God that angers me.

Blasphemy? Not really.

More like authenticity. More like the God I know.

A Tiny Love Story in One Hundred Words

After my child's brain tumor diagnosis, I suddenly found myself in a mixed marriage. I chose the church of medical journals and second opinions; he went for ancient Jewish texts and amulets. As we hurtled through trauma, we battled our gods on different pages of the same book, both leading to the same hopeful ending. We learned the hard truth that trial drugs for brain tumors sometimes carry the same survival statistics as blessings and prayers. Marital compromise was once just about Netflix and plate patterns. It became finding peace in the differing theologies of survival. The theologies of hope.

WOMAN

The roles we play throughout life are varied and unique. For the most part, I have moved seamlessly between them, shifting from mother to friend to wife. Somewhere along the line, it's easy to lose sight of our own identity.

When my son relapsed, I stopped reading fiction. I also stopped writing. I felt like I had been launched into another world, again. I was waiting for the proverbial shoe to drop, and while that happened, I turned into someone I didn't recognize.

I had my body cut up. I had already lost my breasts, and soon after, I lost my ovaries and uterus. I watched my son struggle with tumors that waited to return or just bided their time, and through it all, I lost myself a bit.

But I like to think I came back.

I saw my reflection change over the years. I watched as my needs were put to the side, my wants and desires placed second—not because anyone forced me, but because I simply forgot. Forgot that before cancer came into my life, I was a woman with interests outside of reading medical journals and MRI reports. At one point I was a Neil Gaiman fan, a reader of Stephen King, and a collector of all things fandom. I was a five-time C-section warrior, a woman with ideas that went beyond just kids and medicine and fighting to survive.

I came back, but I was different. I started running—a task that was never even on my list, let alone a bucket list. I found new friends. I raised half a million dollars for a charity I believed in, and I ran in five half-marathons. I wasn't the woman I started out as—I was changed.

These are the chapters about me. They are the essays that remind me who I was before, during, and after the years of breast cancer and brain tumors. Like most people, I'm a work in progress and still redefining myself—rediscovering who I am daily.

But I'm reading again. And writing. And embracing whoever appears in my ever-changing mirror each day.

Scars

My scars are everywhere, faded to white over the years, but still there.

The long white line that stretches across my belly where five kids kicked and screamed their way into the world.

The raised blotch on my knee from the paintball gun episode in tenth grade.

The tiny mark on my lower back—the last remnants of a potentially tragic accident involving a crochet hook, a bus, and a new understanding of velocity.

The evidence of the chicken pox pustule on my neck that I scratched, and the shingles that showed up years later after three days of having too much fun with friends.

The muffler burn that forced me to tell my parents I had been on the back of a motorcycle.

They are everywhere. Like lightning bolts that tell a story of my life.

There are others, though, just below the surface.

The scars I carry from the girls in middle school, whose words somehow still echo when I look in the mirror. The scars from my eleventh-grade math teacher, whose conde-scending voice I still hear every time I have to do a simple equation. The scars that bleed again and again when I see my daughter struggling in school, or my son not getting on the team.

They are the scars that define my movements, guide my words, influence my choices.

You can't see them; you wouldn't even know they are there. But they have shaped my heart, my mind, my body.

I used to hide them. Ashamed of what they were, ashamed of my weaknesses and frailties. Now, I know better.

They are the war marks of a life lived—Hamlet's heart-ache and the natural shocks that flesh is heir to.

The older I get, the more scars I accumulate. I'm still getting them. Still feeling new stings that I know will leave a mark and change the way I live my life, or speak to friends, or view the world.

Sometimes, my scars set me on an entirely new course, and then they are more like stamps on a passport. Gateways I've traveled through, sights I've seen, snapshots of moments that somehow changed me. Some more subtle than others.

I've been thinking about these scars I carry, and wonder-ing about the ones I've inflicted on others without realizing it. Maybe when I wasn't sensitive enough. Or when I was simply cruel.

That's really all we are, I guess. Far from perfect. Far from pristine. As citizens of the world, we are scarred, and marked, and changed, and continually transforming. Our hurts and our pains are absorbed, and as time moves on, we have to choose how they will heal. Will they fester and blister and consume us with rage or thoughts of revenge? Or will they fade and become a part of us, transforming us, making us better as a result of our flaws?

My scars are everywhere. I see them in the mirror. I feel them in my soul. They are the roadmap of my life.

And I embrace them.

Paint Your Pain

"Paint your pain," my friend said, and I sort of rolled my eyes. Because the idea of painting *that* was a bit overwhelming. Truth be told, the very idea of even *painting* seemed like asking a lot. I'm not an artist. I don't know how to approach a canvas. I don't know about mixing colors on a palette and whatnot.

But still, I sat with her in her small studio and explored what I could try to create. My pain was vast. I could start with my childhood. I could paint my middle-school years. I could paint my breast cancer. My child's brain tumor diagnosis. My recent hysterectomy. The list was long, and the idea of putting everything onto a canvas was too great. My mind was a mess, and the more I tried to put everything together into one image, the more inadequate I felt.

Great, I thought. I could add "inadequate" to the list.

I started to think in terms of colors. If my pain picture had a shade, I knew it wasn't going to be bright. I picked up the brush and created a gray background with swirls of black mixed in. Soon, the idea came to me—the presentation of my pain—and I was painting. My insecurities fell to the side and I worked on my canvas, focusing all my emotions and energy from the previous few years onto the small square in front of me.

It took some time, but eventually, I finished it. The grays and blacks mixed with brighter shades of gold and red. The images were mine, and they told a story that was unique to my experience. My painting mirrored the process it took to create it. It was raw. It was real. It revealed a truth that I knew all along about how I deal with my pain, how I share it, how I hide it, and how I hold it at bay.

I was proud of it in an embarrassed sort of way. After all, I'm not a great artist. I didn't expect that much.

But I also didn't expect what happened the next day.

The day after I "painted my pain," I woke up early, went for a run, and started my day feeling physically lighter than I had in weeks. It wasn't a subtle change, mind you. It was powerful. The coffee wasn't as bitter, my mind was a bit clearer, and my energy was higher than it had been in a long time. I didn't think it was a coincidence.

John Sarno, an expert on chronic pain, talks about how pent-up emotions find their way to other parts of your body. That back pain? Probably childhood trauma. Pain, as John Green once wrote, demands to be felt. And if we believe that physical pain can be healed with casts, braces, and analgesics, then the emotional pain we carry around sometimes needs more than just a good conversation with a well-trained therapist. Sometimes it needs a physical place to go to. And sometimes we need the physical act of putting it there.

Like death and taxes, pain is one of those sureties in life. My pain is always with me, shaping me into who I am, guiding my choices and my experiences. Painting it—giving it a physical home—took some of its power and confined it to a twelve-by-ten canvas. It's still there, hanging in my closet where I can see it occasionally. A symbol of its constancy in my life.

"Paint your pain," she said. And I did, in blacks and grays and reds and golds. I thought I was painting with the colors of hurt and anguish. Of tragedy and sorrow.

I didn't realize I was painting with the colors of strength.

And in the end, I created a portrait of resilience.

In the end, I painted myself.

Amanda Palmer Saved My Boobs

No, really.

She doesn't know this, but she is directly responsible for my boobs.

I know that's a heavy responsibility, and I know that my relationship with Amanda Palmer is solely based on reading her Tweets and Facebook posts. I know she doesn't even realize what she has done, but here I am announcing it to the world: Amanda f-ing Palmer saved my boobs.

I should probably support her Patreon.

It happened a year after my mastectomy and three months after my son's brain tumor diagnosis. She was nine months pregnant and participating in a living art installation at the New York Public Library. She was standing in front of the library, naked but covered in body paint, promoting children's literacy. I was completely covered up, hiding a year's worth of tamoxifen and depression-induced weight gain, reading medical journals and Wikipedia articles.

I was a year into reconstruction. The mastectomy was supposed to just be prophylactic but—surprise!—three invasive tumors were sneakily hidden from all the images taken prior. What with all the "You're so lucky!" comments, I was a bit of a mess. I had my final reconstruction surgery scheduled. Two weeks before that surgery, I was in the hospital with my youngest son, finding out he had a brain tumor. While scheduling his craniotomy and looking for specialists, I had stopped the tamoxifen and canceled my surgery.

Ain't nobody got time for that.

I really didn't care about my breasts at that point and figured I was fine with the Frankenboobs. I wasn't planning on going topless in the foreseeable future. My boobs would forever be covered in tank tops, T-shirts, or hoodies. I was fine.

And then Amanda Palmer showed up at the New York Public Library, sword in hand, nine months pregnant, confident, and secure. The artwork on her body was incredible, so I watched the behind-the-scenes video of how it was done. And that's when it hit me.

I had forgotten what breasts looked like.

I watched that video a few times, creepily—I know—looking at Amanda Palmer's nine-months-pregnant breasts. I was shocked that I had forgotten what I used to look like (though granted, I'm pretty sure her nine-months-pregnant breasts looked way better than mine ever did). And for the first time since my diagnosis, and in the shattering aftermath of my son's diagnosis, I wanted to get them back. I called my plastic surgeon the next day and rescheduled the final surgery.

At the time, I think I was motivated by the sheer awe of forgetting what a breast with nipples looked like. Not the prosthetic foobs I had sported since that surgery a year and a bit prior. But I recognized that it was also the first time I'd made a decision to do something solely for myself. To take an active role in the "cancer journey" everyone talks about that I hated.

I could have been fine without nipples—tattooed or otherwise—but in the depth of chaos, I wanted to get some semblance of myself back. I wanted to get my boobs back. I know the questions this decision raised: Aren't I more than my breasts? Why did something so superficial become so important to me—a rallying point for what I felt was a return to normalcy? Why did I even care? I'm not even sure I know why. And there are so many women who have a mastectomy and just continue without reconstruction at all.

I've thought about this for a while. Looking back, years later, I remember watching Amanda Palmer, confident in all her glory, not giving a rat's ass about being naked, or pregnant, or painted, or anything. Maybe I was looking for that.

The day after that surgery, I was convinced I had made an error and that I would never be myself. That I was fooling myself into thinking I could ever go back and erase the whole year.

I was right. I couldn't. And no, even as I finished up the reconstruction process, I was not about to escape the insecurity that comes from having internal prosthetic breasts. I would always have those scars. But going through with the final surgery did allow me to close the door a little bit more, crossing my surgeon off the list of doctors I hopefully would never need to see again.

So even though she doesn't know it, Amanda Palmer saved my boobs. Well, brought them closer to what they were before they tried to kill me. They will never be the same, no question, but in some way, that sword she wielded on the steps of the library filled me with power and strength to take back another piece of my broken body.

I am woman, fake breasts and all.

Illness and the English Language

The following essay by my daughter is a must-read for any-one who has ever had to confront a new world filled with new vocabulary. While I might be a bit close to the source here, I think this powerful essay will speak to others as well.

"Cancer" is a part of the daily vocabulary at my house. Some families introduce dictionary words of the day in an effort to color the vocabularies of their households. My family has medical terms. They pop up in conversations as commonly as words like "chores" or "homework." We don't try to cover them up with false names or platitudes. We spit cancer out like a watermelon seed, firmly and carefully articulated.

"Mastectomy" was a big addition. I remember when I learned that word because I googled it and couldn't sleep for a week. Soon, words like "Trileptal" and "craniotomy" also joined the ranks of our ever-growing family vocabulary.

Translation: my mother was diagnosed with breast cancer in 2014. One year later, my brother had a seizure and shortly after was diagnosed with a brain tumor. He was eight.

211

Accepting that someone in your family has cancer, comes in stages, like the disease itself. And each stage comes with new definitions of terms you once thought you knew.

We all know what "shock" is. But "shock" took on a new meaning for my family and me when it was associated with the possibility of invasive breast cancer. "Shock" went from a word describing the Oscar outcomes to a word that denoted a sudden, irreversible change in our ordinary lives.

Even a simple word like "dinner" took on a new meaning for us. Because in the throes of hospital stays and recoveries, dinner didn't mean home-cooked meals from Mom. Dinner was foil-covered, preprepared ziti with a side of cold soup. "Dinner" was the way my community expressed their concern and support for my family when they were not able to do anything else.

I sometimes think my family should write their own "Dictionary for the Afflicted" to comfort those who feel alone in this process of learning new, uncomfortable words. We alone know that "grueling" reaches a whole new level when it is associated with an eight-hour surgery to extract a brain tumor, and that "waiting," a word usually associated with boredom, is in fact the most painful word in the English language.

I guess my family perfectly encapsulates the ever-changing nature of the English language. Words have different meanings to different people. For some, "benign" might be a textbook term, but for us, it's a real part of our daily lives. And only we understand how the word "positive" can actually be negative when it is associated with oncology.

The new words and meanings flowed seamlessly into our daily dialogue. We learned to eliminate the stigma of illness, not for some noble cause or higher ground, but for ourselves. We did it out of necessity. We needed to be open with each other to create a space for humor and lightness in a state that was anything but that.

And it worked. My mother's daily reminders for my brother to take his tumor medication usually came out in the same breath as her reminder to the rest of us to eat our breakfasts. In our family, "Trileptal" and "diazepam" were as common as "orange juice" and "cornflakes," and my brother appeared all the more normal for it.

We spoke about the hard things, like scars and reconstruction. But we also spoke about the good things. For a kid recovering from a brain tumor, Disney World lived up to its name as the happiest place on Earth, a perfect foil to the hospitals and doctors' offices.

Even the little things were exciting. Never underestimate the power of a hand-knit hat for a bedridden kid who is concealing a scar.

During this time, I liked to think that every addition to our dictionary was a step toward recovery, and in a way, a step closer to normalcy. That in some way, codifying these new words and meanings would help my family make sense of our predicament. Every question would be easily located in an index. We would never be at a loss for words.

But the process of dealing with familial illness doesn't work out as neatly as I had hoped. There is no mathematical equation for achieving equilibrium or returning to "the good old days." You learn as you go, redefining and sharpening terms to fit your new vocabulary.

People used to marvel at my family's ability to move on, as if we were expected to retreat into our hospital wards and wallow for weeks. But we chose to define the words that were thrown at us instead of allowing them to define us.

My family was lucky. Cancer, I guess, didn't win this time, and its versatility surely faded as we threw the word around with no reverence, equating it with all the other nouns in the dictionary. Although we had lived it, we didn't fear it.

Despite all the pain, getting through illness has its upsides too.

Some words, like "victory," become even sweeter.

Twelve Days to Live

It turns out that I have around twelve more days to live.

This was my final assessment after going online to research the symptoms that started plaguing me almost immediately after I waded in some stagnant water.

Stiff neck, headache, fever.

It could have been just a cold, true. But no. After an exhaustive two-minute search on Google, it became clear that I had the deadly brain-eating parasite *Naegleria fowleri*.

It didn't matter that in the last ten years, only thirty-five people in the United States have ever contracted this disease. It didn't matter that technically I didn't *swim* in the waters that might have contained the microscopic bug. Google was pretty clear, and so was SymptomChecker.com. I was going to die.

I gently broke the news to my husband.

He took it well. After all, he is the king of Google diagnoses. Leg cramp? Must be a blood clot. Eye twitch? Check for a worm living behind your cornea. Freckle? It's a melanoma. End stage, by the looks of it.

If anything, the ease of access to information on the internet has made everyone an expert in the medical field. Doctors are no longer the enlightened healers who know everything. Just a click away is the diagnosis I need to justify taking a skydiving trip and going off my diet.

I imagine this information is crippling to hypochondriacs and worst-case-scenario junkies. There must be whole groups of people harassing their doctors, convinced they have the latest rare disease. It's probably what's driving my insurance premiums up each year.

It isn't just medicine, though. Virtually every profession has a corresponding website that can make anyone an expert in the field, with virtually no training. With a simple search, I can dole out accounting information like a pro. I can find all the symbols and themes of *The Scarlet Letter* without ever cracking open the book. I can argue about the dangers of the Common Core curriculum and why Teach for America is destroying our schools. And don't even get me started on whatever hot topic legal drama is currently playing out in the news and on Twitter. I'm practically a lawyer.

You know what they say about a little knowledge.

I can't really say whether it's all bad. It just changes the worldwide playing field a bit. Now it isn't about what you know, it's about what you choose to *filter*. The knee-jerk reaction people have when they read about some new Facebook privacy violation and post it blindly because it sounds true is the same thing that happens when medical morons search up their symptoms on Google. Because if it's in print, it *must* be true.

Of course, I never do that. I even have Snopes saved as a favorite.

Except for this.

Because my neck hurts. And I was in stagnant water. And clearly, I have some brain-eating parasite.

4:30 a.m.

Here's what happens when I have to drive at 4:30 in the morning out in the mountains and forests of upstate New York.

I start to freak out.

It happens slowly. Since I'm alone, I think about the people who might be hiding in the forest surrounding the winding road I'm traveling on. It's an eleven-minute ride from my house to the highway, and even with SiriusXM blasting, I am counting the seconds.

And then, at the first deserted intersection, there's a car.

Who could possibly be driving at 4:30 a.m.? And why are they following me? I speed up, he speeds up. I slow down, his brights blind me. Is it a cop? If it is, there's no way I am stopping. It could just be a random car with lights attached to it that the psycho behind the wheel uses to pull over unsuspecting drivers at 4:30 a.m.

So yeah, no.

If those lights start spinning and I hear sirens, I'm flooring it. Cavorting deer and skunks be damned.

I realize it must be a serial killer. Even though I'm also a random driver out at 4:30 a.m., I know that *I'm* safe. That means that driver number two is clearly *un*safe.

I glance at Waze, glowing warmly from my phone. No other Wazers online. Obviously. Who would be out at 4:30 a.m.?

The car behind me speeds up and illegally passes me. I don't see anyone in the front seat. Probably because there is no one driving the car. It's a ghost car. No question.

And that's when it hits me that to get to the highway, I need to pass the haunted house.

There is a legit haunted house on the road that I pass virtually every day when I am staying in the area. It's abandoned and falls further and further into disrepair each year. And each year that I come to this wilderness, I swear I will explore it. But I haven't yet.

So now, at 4:30 a.m., I know that whatever is living in that house will no doubt make an appearance in the middle of the road as I pass. And by the way, I'm using the word "living" in the loosest sense of the word. Probably a woman dressed in black rags, holding her hands high, blocking the road. Pale white face. Large bloody grin. No pulse.

I start looking for the serial-killer-ghost-police dude. His taillights have long since pulled away from my field of vision.

I switch the radio station from The Pulse to On Broadway. Music from *The Phantom of the Opera* is playing. Great. I switch to Howard Stern. It's just the news. Not that funny. I'm passing the house soon.

I concentrate on the road in front of me. Not the forest. Not the creepy house looming out of the corner of my eye. Not the movement I swear I see in the forest.

I just look straight ahead.

Why is there so much fog? What is it with the mountains at night?

And then, I see lights. I never realized how comforting a Walmart sign can be at 4:30 in the morning. But there it is, shining like the break of day. The entrance to the highway is right around the corner. I stop scanning on Sirius and settle back on The Pulse. (Great station there, by the way.) I get on the highway and get comfortable for the two-hour drive ahead of me. A drive with no ghosts, no creepy ladies, no haunted houses.

And there, on the side of the road, a little off the exit, is the ghost-serial killer-cop dude. With a state trooper.

Hah. Should've stayed with me instead of racing off.

Wimp.

Coffee Names

Whenever I go to Starbucks, I make up a name. The workers are always so nice, so smiling and cheerful, when they ask my name. I used to think I was unique in this, but then I saw a guy who gave his name as "Evil."

Of course, I try to keep my coffee personas within the realm of reality, and so I have been all sorts of java drinkers.

Interestingly, when I first started giving out fake names, I always stuck to names that started with the letter *A*. I guess it was a familiarity thing. I've been Ally, Amy, Abbie, Ariel, and Andromeda. But I soon branched out into more elaborate-sounding names.

Josephine, Emmaline, Harriet.

Harriet was a tough one. So was Mabel. Astrid got me a funny look (though Andromeda didn't even get a double-take). I was Luna, but not Hermione (too obvious, I thought). And I was Ginny.

It's a stupid little thing, but it makes me smile to have a grande latte with the name "Sienna" emblazoned in black sharpie on the side for everyone to see. It adds another layer to the anonymity of the coffeehouse, I guess. Now, even though you think you know me, you're just so far from who I am. I look around and see all the Mikes and Annas, Peters and Amys, and I'm sipping from my "Farrah" cup, or maybe Cleo. Or Anastasia. And suddenly, I am someone else.

I can't figure out why there is a difference between a Eugene and a John, a Martha and an Andrea. There is something to the names we live with, and whether we become our name or the name shapes us, our entire persona is wrapped up in that name.

Are you a Candy? A Trixie? Definitely the cheerleaders in high school. Are you Elmer the AP Science student, or Elmer the quarterback? More likely the former. In that split second of meeting someone and asking the all-important "What's your name?" question, there is a quick judgment. It's the difference between Eugene and Flynn Rider.

In Starbucks, I try a name on for size, see how it fits, watch the reaction of the cashier as he asks for the spelling ("That's Quathrynn, with a *Q* not a *K*"), and look for some flicker in his eye that tells me he knows. That there's no way that's my name. That I'm a fraud. I'm not Astrid, or Penelope, or Barbara.

But that never happens. I guess because somewhere in Starbucks training, employees are taught to just smile and write the name, whatever it is. That's why for every one of my lame monikers, there are probably a couple thousand Tony Starks.

So last week, I sat down with my "Tina" cup and was joined by a "Brad." He had long, grungy hair and short black boots. Of course, his name was Brad. And since he thought I was Tina, I figured I'd just play along.

We compared laptops. Talked writing. I threw myself into the Tina role. What would a Tina be like? What would she say? How would she act?

For a while there I was pulling it off. Even *I* believed my name was Tina.

And then he said this: "By the way, my name's not really Brad. It's Henry."

I laughed and thanked him for the writing advice ("Get rid of all your adverbs." Thanks, Henry), grabbed my "Tina" cup, and took off. The sociology experiment complete.

I never told him that I wasn't Tina, but I have seen him a few more times at that Starbucks. He's been Max, and Sam, and Joe. Never Henry. But I've never been Tina again either, so I am sure he knows that I'm playing the same little game. I wonder if he knew all along.

But that's okay. After all, I have all day to be myself. At least for a few minutes in Starbucks, I get to be whoever I want.

I think he gets that too.

Whatever his name is.

This is Neil Gaiman We're Talking About Here

In a few days, I am going to meet Neil Gaiman.

As excited as I was when I first volunteered to work at his book signing, I am now, a week before the event, completely panic-stricken.

I mean, this is *Neil Gaiman* we are talking about.

I keep going over the scenario. He walks in, I say "hi." Maybe I'm the coffee runner. Maybe I'm the bouncer. Who knows? I haven't received my job description yet. But that moment when I get to say "hi" is killing me. I can't be too aloof because then I'll seem like a snob. But if I'm too effusive, then I'm just a crazed fangirl.

I don't think there is any way I can get out of this looking good.

I mean, this is Neil *Gaiman* we're talking about.

Of course, I have prepared.

I started my "I'm going to meet Neil Gaiman" crash diet (it's slowly working). I have my requisite black T-shirt in honor of his trademark duds. I have my stack of Gaiman stuff for him to sign: a book for my nephew, a Coraline doll for my daughter, my newly purchased *Make Good Art* book. Plus his recent novel, *The Ocean at the End of the Lane.*

But as a fan, I think I might be pathetic.

See, I've seen Gaiman fans that put me to shame. I don't have quotes from *American Gods* tattooed across my shoulders. I haven't even read *Good Omens.* I watched the movie version of *Coraline* before reading the novel. And I skimmed one of the chapters of *The Graveyard Book* because I was starting to get bored.

So I'm not a die-hard fan. But I am a fan nonetheless.

There is something about Neil Gaiman that is inspiring. For some reason, when I listen to his speeches and snippets of his interviews, when I follow him on Twitter and read his blog, he seems so . . . accessible. Here's a guy who is living the writer's dream, who loves what he does and wants other people to love it as well.

I have never sensed an air of pretension about it.

Granted, I could be way off base here. It's possible that maybe, just maybe, he's a jerk.

But I don't think that's the case.

So why am I so nervous about meeting Neil Gaiman? I mean, I don't think he is so nervous to meet me.

I think it's because I've been thinking about this for so long that when I'm finally there, it will be such a cosmic letdown that I'll just feel like an idiot. I once met Billy Joel at a hotel on the beach. He was playing a concert that night with Elton John, and though I wasn't going to the concert, I pretended I was and spoke to him for a few minutes.

Nice guy, by the way.

But bottom line, even though it was Billy freakin' Joel, he was just a guy. A guy who sings really well and plays piano.

And Neil Gaiman, he's just a guy who writes well.

But, no.

I mean, this is *Neil Gaiman* we're talking about here.

Pass the rice cakes. I have a few more pounds to go.

Meeting Neil

I came to Neil Gaiman in a backwards sort of way. A student of mine, Alex, brought *American Gods* to class and told me I had to read it. I, of course, took the book, thanked him, and proceeded to *not* read it. It sat on my bookshelf. Alex asked me numerous times, and each time, I said that I hadn't gotten around to it. I might have lied at some point and said I had started it, but the truth was, no. It was still there on my shelf. Alex eventually graduated, and the book collected dust for two more years.

And then *The Graveyard Book* came out. It sounded cool, and so I bought it and read it in one night. I loved it. I loved it so much that I convinced my ninth-grade English class that they should read it as well.

Of course, if you read *The Graveyard Book*, you're going to want to read more of Neil Gaiman's work. And lucky for me, there on my bookshelf was Alex's copy of *American Gods*.

Almost three years after it was given to me, I finally read it. And I was hooked.

Here's the thing about Neil Gaiman. If you follow him on Twitter, if you read his blog, if you like him on Facebook, you fall into this bizarre comfort zone. You feel like he's your friend. He's approachable. He's actually talking to you. My relationship with Neil, one-sided as it was, grew over the years. So when I had the chance to work at one of his book signings and meet the man I had followed for years, I jumped at the chance.

I also readied myself. I knew that my perception of my relationship with Neil Gaiman went as far as reading his tweets and updates. While he had a tremendous effect on me and my writing, it didn't work both ways. I knew there would not be this instant friendship, this camaraderie born of tweets and random likes. So going in, I was prepared.

But here's what I wasn't prepared for.

I couldn't hang out with him before the signing because I was running odd jobs in the crowd, but I did get to see him for a few seconds after his short speech. I think our conversation went something like this:

ME: Oh my gosh, it's Neil Gaiman, right here in front of me.

NEIL: Oh my gosh, it is.

Yeah. That went well.

But later, as he signed more than eight hundred books for fans who had stood in line for hours, I was able to sit a few feet away from him and sort of watch the interactions.

If you haven't met Neil Gaiman fans, you need to know that they are really dedicated. Insanely dedicated. Tattoos and paintings and "naming their children for characters he created" dedicated.

I am definitely not in their league.

I was able to talk to many of them, and I created my own little psychological analyses. I would look at their clothes and who they were with, and I could guess what they brought for him to sign.

I knew who the Sandman people were, the *American Gods* people, the *Blueberry Girl* types, and the Graveyard Bookers. Some were a bit scary, true, but everyone was there, waiting for hours, to get some sort of connection to Neil Gaiman.

And, incredibly, as he signed each book that was passed in front of him, I noticed that Gaiman made it a point to look each and every fan right in the eye. He gave them that moment of complete connection that they were looking for. Even if it was for a second, even if he looked back at the book, he made sure that every single fan got that contact.

They felt seen.

I watched this from my vantage point three feet away (at that point, I was directing fans to the exit), and I realized that the original connection I had felt to Neil Gaiman was not just a clever internet marketing trick. He actually believed it. Far from being this arrogant bestseller who wrote from an ivory tower, he was right there with the fans, saying "Thank you" and "It's nice to meet you" and "Yes, please tell me about your dog" and "Wow, what a beautiful gift—my portrait made of pasta and jelly beans." It's why he stays at events, no matter how long, until the last fan leaves.

I spent eight hours working at the event, and I eventually got to talk to him at the end. He read a letter I'd brought from my husband and took pictures. He signed my books and my daughter's Coraline doll. Our straight-up interaction lasted only a few minutes, but I didn't leave disappointed. I left remarkably contented and happy.

After all, it was like saying "hi" to an old friend.

Thanks, Neil.

Lessons From Stephen

It's Stephen King's birthday this week. Saturday, to be exact.

I've been a Stephen King fan for quite some time now. I picked up *Pet Sematary* when I was in ninth grade. At the time, everyone was passing around V. C. Andrews's *Flowers in the Attic* series. And while incestuous sibling relationships and psychotic grandmothers were interesting, I found that my angst-filled teenage youth craved something much darker. Enter Stephen King.

Pet Sematary was the only book that physically scared me. I was reading it on a Friday night. In one scene, the main character breaks in to a cemetery to exhume his dead son's grave. I was in bed, under my covers, my nose inches from the page. And then, the man finally opens the coffin, looks in to see his poor dead son, and there's this line:

"His head was gone."

I threw the book across the room. Something about that blunt statement scared the absolute bejeezus out of me. It helped that it was late at night, that I was the only one up, that my sister was snoring sporadically. But bottom line, I was scared. And I was hooked.

The Shining came next. To this day, I cannot walk between hedges and not think that they are somehow moving closer to me. Even in Disney World, those happy Mickey and Minnie topiaries seem far more sinister than the smiling tourists realize. I see people posing in front of those leafy effigies at the top of Main Street USA, and I swear I see Mickey's grin extend a bit wider than normal, see his eyebrows furrow. And when did he get teeth?

I grabbed every Stephen King book I could find—an easy thing to do, considering the rate at which he publishes—and since I was a bit late to the party, I had a lot to choose from. I read *Misery* in one night, finishing it at 4:30 a.m. It remains the only book I ever read in one sitting. None of the books in the Harry Potter series even managed to do that. I bought *The Bachman Books* and read those. Picked up *Salem's Lot* and discovered vampires the way they were meant to be discovered. "Cujo" became the catchword for every mangy mutt that wandered without a leash around the boardwalk where I grew up ("Stay away from that cute pup—it's a Cujo."). And now, whenever I go through the Lincoln Tunnel in New York, all I can imagine is Larry Underwood's terror-filled walk through the pitch-dark, body-filled tunnel in *The Stand*.

As I searched for King, I didn't discriminate. I loved *The Eyes of the Dragon*, my precursor to all things fantasy and no doubt the reason for my Harry Potter obsession years later. His collections of short stories were my favorites. *The Mist* was one of those stories everyone tried to rehash at camp, but no one could ever tell it as good as the King, and I would just roll my eyes and roast my marshmallows. *Firestarter* convinced me that the government was hiding all knowledge of paranormal activity in this country, and that more importantly, there was some way I could harness it for myself.

But in tenth grade I read *The Body*, the story that probably changed my life. That was when I decided I wanted to be a writer. I loved the story so much that I convinced a friend to come with me on an adventure. We took our bikes and followed the railroad tracks near her home in upstate New York while I told stories and imagined myself looking for the body of Ray Brower. It's remarkable that we weren't killed by the vagrants we passed along the way.

As a fledgling writer at age sixteen, I quickly became an arrogant critic. I was an authority on the writer who consumed most of my reading time but who could clearly use some pointers from me, a brilliant teenager. I was kind of like that kid in *Apt Pupil*. But I wasn't holding anyone hostage or cutting myself in private.

My arrogance didn't last too long. I thought I was a Jedi when, in truth, it was too soon for me to leave Dagobah. With each of his books, I learned more and more. I read about King's influences. I mimicked his style. I referenced his work in my papers for school (always met with a terse "this is not an author of literary merit" comment from the teacher). My college thesis was titled "Horror and Literature."

Take *that*, high-school lit teacher.

As I grew, so did King. My tastes changed. His writing changed. My obsession tapered off and was replaced by other authors, but he was always there, in the periphery. I can't claim to have read all his books—I never picked up *The Dark Tower*, I didn't finish *Hearts in Atlantis*, and *Under the Dome* is still on my shelf waiting—but I can't deny his influence on my writing and reading tastes.

And the lessons I have learned from him go far beyond staying away from sewers or realizing that the past is obdurate. They are the lessons I keep in my writing toolbox. Lessons I pull out when I write and teach. And lessons that my daughter is just learning as she picks up her first Stephen King books. Lessons summed up by one of my favorite quotes: ". . . keep smiling. Get a little rock and roll on the radio, and go toward all the life there is with all the belief you can find and all the truth you can muster. Be true. Be brave. Stand. All the rest is darkness."

Happy birthday, Mr. King, from one of your (mostly) constant readers.

Old ... er

Yes, it's my birthday. The anniversary of when I showed up in this world and a nice reminder that I'm still here. Also, a nice reminder that I'm older and that much closer to *not* being here.

Cue the narcissistic, self-pitying music.

I know they always say "Age is just a number!"—which is really one of the dumbest things ever. That's like saying "Words are just letters!" or "Obnoxious finger gestures are just phalanges!" Obviously age is a number, but it isn't "just" a number. It places you in some category. In a generation. In a checkbox on the AARP website. It's way more than just a number. It's an identity.

I used to have this theory that while everyone ages at the same rate, most people hit a particular age and then psychologically just stay there. Sometimes they hit that mark way before they reach that physical age. Those were the kids in high school who were like thirty-five-year-olds when they were seventeen. Or now, even people younger than me sometimes seem older because they were *always* like fifty-year-olds. And the opposite is true as well. Some people are tragically trapped as five-year-olds, behaving as such when they are pushing forty.

So even though it's my birthday and I'm older, I don't really feel older. True, I've changed physically. I'm noticing gray hairs and lines on my face. It's harder to lose weight and easier to gain it. My knees sometimes hurt. But I still feel like I can cartwheel down a hallway, and there are times I definitely don't act my age. I'm always balancing that feeling with the very real fear of looking like one of those older people trying to look young and cool. Or like I'm perpetually in the middle of a really bad midlife crisis, and none of my friends have the heart to say that I look ridiculous.

It's great that it's my birthday, and that I'm alive and all that, but at the same time, I'm still in shock when I think about how many years I've been here. I'm even more shocked that at the same time, it doesn't seem like so many years. I wish I knew exactly when that transference occurred—the moment when the years sped up and time suddenly seemed a lot shorter than it had before. Or that moment when my backache switched from "I must have been holding the baby wrong" to "Oh my God, it must be cancer."

Actually, I can pinpoint the exact day that last one happened, but still.

I always get philosophical on my birthday, but the truth is, it really isn't as big a deal as I make it. The melancholy mood, the pensive stare, and the pondering on mortality quickly give way to the cake and ice cream and homemade cards sprinkled through the day. And Facebook becomes a virtual drive-through surprise party, with hundreds of friends dropping by to say "Happy Birthday" on their way down their newsfeeds.

It's true, I'm older. My kids remind me of that with funny cards and good-natured jokes. My younger ones were literally born in a different century, making the divide that much more surreal. But even so, regardless of all the annoyances and aggravations that getting older brings, the alternative is definitely not an option I'm rushing toward.

So happy birthday to me—another year older, another year grateful to sit and write a birthday post from a mature, adult perspective.

Which means I'm still eating that cake and ice cream. And maybe playing a round of musical chairs.

Cheating

I was at dinner with friends when someone asked me about cheating in school. She wanted to know the moral implications of cheating—what it says about a person who would copy someone else's work. And are there different levels of cheating? Is copying someone's homework as bad as copying from someone's test? If everyone is cheating, does that make a difference?

Of course, it isn't something I am that familiar with. Me cheat? Never.

I'll give you a moment to get over that statement.

Truth is, and I know this will shock you, I have cheated in school. I've copied someone's homework when I didn't do mine. At the time, I don't think I felt I was crossing any moral line that put me on some cosmic lower level of society. I just needed to get a grade, and besides, the teacher never read the homework anyway. They were just minor infractions.

But then there was this one time.

It was June. End of the school year. And I was walking to school on the morning of my Chemistry Regent. In case you aren't familiar with them, New York State requires these end-of-the-year subject exams called Regents. I think they still give them. Anyway, I usually took the city bus to get to school, but that day I decided to walk the twenty blocks instead.

For the record, I had studied for my Chem Regent. I even had a tutor (who, years later, became my brother-in-law). I wasn't really worried about the exam. I only needed to pass.

I had stopped at a corner newsstand to pick up a chocolate bar when I saw it.

There, on the cover of the *New York Post*, were the answers to the Chem Regents. The one I was about to take.

For a moment, I wasn't sure if anyone else could see what I was seeing. I thought I was getting some kind of divine prophecy, right there on the corner of Bedford Avenue. But it was real. The *New York Post* had published the answers to that day's exam as part of an exposé on the rampant cheating on state exams. To prove their point about how easy it was to cheat, they released the answers in advance of the test.

Lucky me.

So now comes the big question. Did I buy the paper that day? And if I did, did I pause before I purchased a copy? Did I wonder about the moral and ethical decision I had to make? Everyone had already seen it. My entire class had seen it. Hell, my entire grade in the state of New York had seen it. I was surprised that my school even gave us the exam that day.

I walked into school and my chem teacher was livid.

"Everyone has the answers!" he yelled.

He was right. The girl sitting next to me had written them all in the hem of her skirt. Another girl had them carved into her pencil.

Where was I in all this? That was the question my friend posed to me yesterday. Is it wrong to cheat even when everyone else is? If the answers to my exam are published on the front page of the newspaper, should I turn away? Or should I level the playing field and join the masses?

I thought about my Chem Regent and about that day on the street when I could have sworn God had given me a gift. And I thought about what was going through my mind that day. What debate did I have with myself? Was that moment a test of my moral fiber?

I really don't think it was, but I still wasn't sure how to answer my friend's questions. After all, I'm not the morality police. And over the years, I have seen good, honest, deeply moral students hand in papers that were plagiarized. I have seen them copy someone else's paper during a test. It's a flaw in the human condition, not necessarily the individual.

So I came up with the worst answer an educator could probably give someone about cheating:

"I really don't care."

Not that I condone cheating, but ultimately, it's the cheater who has to weigh his or her actions. I can give out consequences and speak in my stern, disappointed teaching voice, but deciding on levels of morality—"Is this worse? Does this make it better?"—isn't really something I need to waste time on. When the moment comes, there are lines everyone draws regarding what they will or will not do. Copy a homework assignment? Copy an exam? Steal an exam? Buy a newspaper with the published answers? Where those lines are drawn is what defines an individual.

Like Candide says, "We must all tend our gardens."

I got a ninety-eight on my Chem Regent.

Ten Worst Things to Say to Someone Who Has Had a C-section

I've had five C-sections. Only one of them was "planned." Yes, I labored four times for too many hours, pushed for too many more, and still ended up in the OR having my babies by scalpel. I had three different doctors and two midwives, and I delivered at three different hospitals. At one point in this journey, I joined a rather violent anti-C-section online group. I left after someone posted that they would rather their baby had died than have been born via surgery. I suggested therapy. She suggested I was insensitive and should leave the group.

I did.

It was a moment of clarity for me. It was when I backed off the birthing train, looked at my children, and was able to just say "thank you." This past week though, someone posted the following on an online forum:

"A woman that has a C-section did not educate herself before labor."

I didn't jump into the fray (it was on a cooking forum, which is completely insane by itself), because I knew it was no doubt spoken by someone with zero experience. But as someone who went through so many surgeries, did the research, and tried all the herbs, the positions, the midwives, the doctors, the doulas, the breathing, the hypnosis, the castor-oil labor inductions—I think I am in a position to give some words of advice to those who lack the same experience but continue to offer advice to those on the other side. I'm all for VBACs and natural births, mind you. But there has to be some pragmatism at play that, for some reason, disappears whenever this topic comes up.

So here you go. Your friend just had a baby and it was delivered by C-section. When you go and visit her in the hospital, keep the following in mind. These are things you should never say to a woman who has given birth by C-section. These were all said to me at one point, by the way, and at the time, I died a little. But now, older and wiser, I can roll my eyes and confidently say, "You are a moron," even to the most educated of my friends.

1. *"Oh, you are so lucky! I wish I could have a C-section!"* Yeah, so you're pretty much ignorant. I know all you are thinking about is the convenience of scheduling a birth, and maybe missing the hours of labor, but seriously, no one in their right mind would ever wish for major abdominal surgery just days before having a newborn placed into her care. While you can't walk. Or turn over. Or, sometimes, breathe.

2. *"Have you considered a home birth for the next one?"* Thanks! I'll look into that. Home birth! Great idea. Yes. I did consider it. But once you have a C-section that saves both your life and the life of your baby, you tend to want to focus on surviving more than on the experiential aspect of the whole thing. This comment is always made by someone who does not care what went into the decisions prior to the C-section. They just care that you had one. Don't assume that the surgery was frivolous. It isn't always. And suggesting a home birth for someone who could be high risk is just unwise.

3. *"I heard you had an epidural. Once you start down that path, you're pretty much guaranteed a C-section."* I love this one. You can swap out epidural for any sort of pain medication, by the way. It's the martyr line. The one that implies that if you would have just held out a little longer . . .

Sigh.

Here's what I learned: every labor is different. And your four-hour labor is not the same as my twenty-six-hour labor. And for the record, the main side effect of an epidural is not a C-section, it's pain relief. It can also, as in my case, make the labor speed up. So take your "I didn't have an epidural!" badge, mix it with your granola and wheat germ, and kindly shove it up your ass.

4. *"Did you try a different position?"* I got this gem after giving birth to my son. I pushed for close to three hours. Though a lot of it is fuzzy, I think at a certain point I was hanging from the ceiling. The assumption is always that if I had just tried one more position, the baby would have just flown right out. It isn't always the case.

5. *"I am so sorry for you!"* Why? Because I just gave birth to a beautiful, healthy baby? The correct greeting should really be "Congratulations!" It's a happy event, not a death. It's true, it didn't go as I planned, but give that time. Parenting doesn't go as planned either. Not much in life does. In fact, there is something to be said about learning that you can't control everything when it comes to your kids. I just learned it on the labor floor. It'll hit you when your kid turns three.

6. *"Babies born by C-section develop all sorts of issues. Like learning disabilities. And allergies."* This was brought to my attention by a well-meaning friend who wanted to warn me that I should look for those signs later on in my child's development. Ironically, years later, her kids were pretty much allergic to air and struggling in school. Go figure.

7. *"You live in a state with a high C-section rate."* Yes, that's true. Your point? Should I move? Or again, are you

assuming it was needless? Don't go there. Yes, there are high rates of C-sections in my state, but there are also low rates of infant and maternal mortality. Keep that in mind when you visit your friend.

8. *"It's such a violent way for your child to come into the world."* Hmm . . . Yes, that's true. Giving birth underwater while humming to Enya, surrounded by scented candles—sounds lovely. It's kind of the same vision I had about breast-feeding. I imagined sitting under a tree, wind in my hair, nourishing my baby. The truth? It's painful. It's not "simple." And more often than not, it is almost savage. Childbirth turns the weakest women into Amazonian warlords. I don't think there is one species on the planet that gives birth in peace. (Maybe whales, but even then, it's a *whale*.) Birth is a natural part of life, but don't kid yourself—it's called "labor" for a reason. My C-section is no more violent than a breech birth, or a birth after hours of labor, or even a birth where the baby falls out with seconds to spare.

9. *"Why do you want your child born in a hospital?"* So, first off, see #2 above. Then, consider this: I'd like my kid born in a hospital because there are *doctors* there. And pain-killers. And specialists. So yes, I choose to err on the side of caution. It's why I also vaccinate my kids. Do you want to have that conversation as well?

10. *"You should read this book about childbirth in America."* Someone actually handed me *Silent Knife* a day after my C-section. It was a great read, and it put me in touch with a whole crew of people who preyed on my feelings of inadequacy for failing to have a baby the "natural" way. It educated me, but ultimately, I probably would have been happier with some lighter, more positive reading. Like Stephen King.

So much planning goes into childbirth, and when those plans go awry, it's difficult to recover. I struggled with my birthing experiences for years before ultimately seeing the big picture—that childbirth is not about expectations. It is about the baby. It is about a healthy mom. Stop judging women for how they have their babies and stop making it something much more than it is. The few seconds when my oldest child came into this world do not hold a candle to the years that followed. They do not define her. And they do not define me.

"Do You Wanna Build a Snowman?"

There's nothing like a Disney movie to get you thinking. Have you seen *Frozen* yet? No? You should. It's just fantastic. If I had seen it earlier, I would have written a review. Fortunately, I caught the movie as it was leaving theaters. I'm not going to tell you about the film here (other than that you should see it), but you need to know that it's a movie about relationships, true love, and family. Specifically, sisters.

So this one is for the sisters.

I'm lucky. I have three of them. Though if you asked me years ago, I would have told you it was the worst. We fought all the time. I even recall punching one of my younger sisters. It could have just been a dream though. I remember having that dream often.

I shared a room with two of them (not at the same time, mind you) and was jealous that the youngest one had her own room—a luxury no one else in my family had. My oldest sister was the neat one. She complained that I never made my bed, that my clothes were everywhere, and that I kept her up at night. While it's true that I talked in my sleep, she was a sleepwalker, so I think it balanced out. Her papers were filed and organized. Mine were piled around my desk, crumpled in balls, and stowed under my bed. She studied and did well. I didn't study and got by.

It was clearly a match made in heaven.

By the time she moved out, I was excited for my own room. But before I could even switch beds, my younger sister moved in.

My parents were clever that way.

We were both relatively sloppy and only saw the floor after one of our notorious late-night "let's clean up the room" fests, where we would pile everything in the center of the room and give ourselves ten minutes (maybe five) to put everything away. I usually threw a lot of things on the floor of my closet or under the bed. Next to the old papers. The important thing was that it *looked* clean.

Sibling relationships change over time, and fortunately, my sisters and I have grown closer. I laugh when I think of the fights we had as kids, and more often I remember the fun things we used to do. Like the time my older sister and I put all our stuffed animals on the roof outside our window. Or when my younger sister and I rearranged the entire downstairs while our parents were asleep. I remember teaching my youngest sister how to play a duet on the piano that we called "The Muppet Song," though I am sure it has a real name. Ironic now that I think of it, because she was a far superior piano player even then, when she was five.

We were rarely home as teenagers, spending those years in separate spheres but still together. Always ending our phone conversations or letters with "I love you" or "I miss you" or more often with both. It wasn't something I ever thought twice about.

I always thought that was typical of sisters, but sadly, it isn't. In many cases, people with sisters never get beyond that angry, fighting stage. It follows them into adulthood like a black cloud of jealousy, or resentment, or worse, indifference.

My sisters are my built-in friends, bound by blood, our relationship forged through years of bickering and comforting. We are there for each other, even when we can't physically be present. Through the births of babies, through pain and loss, through marriage and moving, my sisters are on the phone, on Facebook, on Twitter. They call from across miles and across oceans, never feeling as far away as they actually are. We share secrets no one else knows. We share memories created during late-night thunderstorms and rain-soaked boardwalk treks. We grew up on the same foods and pretty much wore the same clothes. Our kids play the same games we invented on endless Saturday afternoons. We cheer each other's successes, mourn each other's losses, commiserate on the bad days, and playfully one-up each other on whatever our pre-coffee morning looked like. Our paths have taken us to different parts of the world, but our bond is still as strong as in those days when we were jumping on beds, rolling our eyes at each other, and slamming doors.

I still miss it though.

None of them has escaped to an ice castle on the top of a mountain, but rest assured, if one of us ever did, the rest would all come running. After all, we're sisters.

And it's been a while since we built a snowman.

Addiction Isn't Real

Philip Seymour Hoffman is dead. Found in his New York apartment with a needle stuck in his arm, pretty much eliminating foul play or any sort of speculation over the cause of death.

He was forty-six years old. He had three kids that were waiting for him at the park with their mother.

And instead, he's dead on the floor of his apartment.

His death took me back to when I heard about River Phoenix and his last hours in the Viper Room. I still have the obituary from *The New York Times*. It was the first time I was so personally affected by a celebrity's death. I was overwhelmed with sadness. It wasn't just that it was River Phoenix, that beautiful man whose face decorated my wall for years. It was his talent, his potential, that was gone. I felt cheated. There was so much I wanted to see him do, so many films I wanted to watch. I mean, he was going to be the next Indiana Jones! It would never happen. It was over.

I also didn't want to believe that he died from an overdose.

"No way! River? He was a vegetarian! Mr. Healthy! It's a lie!"

Of course, it wasn't a lie, but I refused to buy it. At least for as long as I could deny the reports that were all over the news. I didn't want to believe that someone with so much going for him could throw it away like that.

What a waste.

Flash forward and there's another dead talent. True, between River and Philip Seymour Hoffman, there have been quite a number of talented people lost to drugs. But this was something different. This time, for some reason, I found myself back in 1993, remembering River. Feeling that same shock.

Maybe it's because I have a connection to Philip Seymour Hoffman. I met him before he was famous. I ran into him and said, "Hey! Aren't you that guy from *Twister*?" And he said, "Yeah, that's me." And I said, "That's cool. I liked that movie." We spoke for a bit. Nothing major. I didn't ask for an autograph because he wasn't really anybody back then. Plus, I didn't even know his name. He was just some almost-famous guy who grudgingly spoke to me. When he started getting lead roles, that conversation became my little "brush with glory," and it was a cool story I would retell and embellish depending on my audience.

My shock over his death quickly gave way to anger. Anger at the same things from 1993: wasted talent, lost potential, a meaningless death. So I tried to understand his death in the framework of addiction. I read the articles, listened to interviews that likened it to a disease like cancer, but I just wanted to yell, "No! It isn't! Stop making excuses! He chose this!"

That's when I realized I know nothing. A friend of mine put it into perspective for me: "Addiction isn't real," he said, "because you can't fathom it."

It's true. The closest thing to addiction that I know is maybe my "battle" with nail biting. Or knowing that if I walk into a casino with one hundred dollars, I'll walk out in debt. I've gotten drunk at parties, but I'm hardly an alcoholic. I've done stupid things. But I recover. Laugh it off. Hide the pictures.

I don't know what it's like to be alone in an apartment, desperately needing heroin coursing through my veins. I don't know what depths of despair can put someone there or what demons wander through his head, haunting him at every turn. I don't know how someone who seems to have everything can still crave the very thing that will destroy him. I don't understand it.

It isn't real. Not to me. But it most definitely exists. To people who have struggled with this beast, to people who have watched others spiral out of control even after years of being clean—it's real. It's tangible. It's as blatant as a dead man with a needle in his arm.

I don't know Philip Seymour Hoffman to say that I'll miss him. Beyond that one moment, back when he played a nameless character, I know him the way the rest of the world does. A talented actor. A haunted man.

An addict.

And it just leaves me so sad.

O Captain! My Captain!

Robin Williams turned me into a teacher. Turned me on to poetry. Made me want to believe in the power of words and music.

Granted, he didn't write the screenplay for *Dead Poets Society*, but I doubt it could have been told as well with someone else at the helm. And it doesn't really make a difference. Because for me, he will always be the captain.

I was in high school when the movie came out, and my experience with education had been less than stellar. I had teachers who destroyed subjects for me. Teachers who didn't care. I loved writing, and my principal wouldn't let me into the creative writing class. Loved English, but I wasn't allowed to take the AP class. Needless to say, I eagerly awaited the day I could walk away from education forever and settle into some profession that required minimal intellectual aggravation.

And then there was *Dead Poets Society*.

I wanted to be in that school. I was so starved for inspiration, for someone to believe in me, that I would pretend I was one of the boys in the class. I even looked for glasses that matched the ones Robert Sean Leonard wears when he reads from that god-awful guide to poetry at the beginning of the film. After graduation, my friends and I started our own Dead Poets Society. We were in Israel for the year and would escape to random caves and archaeological digs in the middle of the night with a book of poetry and some candles. We climbed the Old City walls at 3 a.m. and stormed the ramparts when everyone else was asleep. One night, we met some strangers, took them with us to our abandoned caves, and asked them to read poetry with us. I still have our poetry book, purchased in a used-book shop that year.

It was remarkable that we even survived. Remarkable that we weren't shot, or entombed, or kidnapped. We were crazy Americans in a foreign country, but we were "sucking the marrow out of life" and enjoying every minute. When we returned to the States, no one believed us. The stories seemed unreal. Too perfect. And they were. At least for the people who kept their fictions on pages or screens. For us, well, those were the realities we wanted, and so we abandoned safety and rules. We made the movie our life. We were Mr. Keating's students.

Stephen King inspired me to write, but Robin Williams was the teacher I had been wishing for. He was the one who could have lit a fire under me in high school, back when all I did was dream of the end of the day. And his example guided me on my first day of work as an English teacher. He was the teacher I wanted to be.

I am keenly aware of how a character can impact a person because my life has always been influenced by books, TV, and movies. When I heard that Robin Williams had died, it knocked the wind out of me. Because my daily choices in my classroom were so influenced by a character he played, I felt like I had lost a mentor. I had lost my captain.

It's too late to write to him and let him know what he did for me. Too late to tell him that he was the one who could always make me laugh. Too late to tell him that his talents spanned generations, that my kids think of him when they think of Peter Pan. That he will always be the nanny everyone wants, the doctor everyone looks for, the DJ we want to hear. That he was the consummate teacher and my captain. Always.

I will miss him, and all the characters that will no longer live through him.

And I'm so sorry I waited to thank him.

> *Exult O shores, and ring O bells!*
> *But I with mournful tread,*
> *Walk the deck my Captain lies,*
> *Fallen cold and dead.*

That One Book

There are two kinds of readers.

The first is that precocious kid who started reading before pre-K. The kid whose parents didn't know what to do when he'd already devoured every book in the (enter grade level) curriculum and needed more. That's the kid who advanced through the steps of literacy from *Goodnight Moon* to *Amelia Bedelia* to *Captain Underpants* to *Narnia*. Books and reading were always a part of his life.

But there is another kind of reader. The kid who never liked reading. When he was in third grade, his parents were concerned that he didn't like to sit down with a good book. That he only wanted to run outside, or build, or play video games. He was the kid who learned about SparkNotes in fifth grade and faked his reading log so he would pass middle-school English. But he became a reader anyway, and more than likely, it was because of one book.

So many people become lifelong readers because of one title. It's their defining book. The one that opened a world to them. J. K. Rowling, John Green, Neil Gaiman, Stephen

King—all of them have written books that launched readers into other works. There are more authors like them. Sometimes it's Jodi Picoult. Sometimes, yes, it's Stephenie Meyer. Sometimes the book is *The Sandman*. It's all that struggling middle schooler needs, and whatever works, let it work.

I was thinking about this when I was tagged in a Facebook status about the books that changed my life. I never answered it, sorry. It was interesting to read other people's lists, though, even though it was probably unfair that I didn't contribute to the trend. I saw classic titles—the Harry Potter books featured prominently—but also some random ones. Comic books and graphic novels made the lists as well. Some people listed the Bible, which is nice and all, but c'mon. There were a few pretentious titles: *Walden*, *The Scarlet Letter*, *Billy Budd* (seriously?). But overall, it was a good list of the gateway books. The ones you need to watch out for. The ones that might lead you down a dangerous path of fiction, lined with dog-eared copies of beloved stories.

I've watched that happen to people who claim they "never read." I've watched people in the grips of their first reader's high after finishing a book, trying to thrust it on anyone who will listen: "You *must* read this book!" I still experience that high sometimes, but there is nothing like the first time. And the more I read, the more critical I become. The more my tastes are refined, the higher I set my standards, and the harder it is to get that new-book excitement.

I'm jealous of those newbies.

But every once in a while, I get a hold of a book that puts me back in that moment. That moment where I read slowly, to savor every page. The book that leaves me wanting more. The book that makes me run to my neighbor's house, thrust it into her hands, and say, "You *must* read this!"

I have a couple titles waiting on my shelf. One of them, I hope, will be that one book. Again.

My Desk

I don't have a desk and it's starting to be a problem.

Granted, I don't think that having one would make me all that more organized and on top of my work. I mean, the idea of having neatly color-coded files placed elegantly in a sturdy drawer rarely ever pans out like the picture in the Ikea catalog. And although I like to think that having a bulletin board with clever-looking pushpins and a ribbon border would simplify the chaos of my invitations, documents, and important appointments, I also know that I would likely fail to *find* the cute pushpins when I needed to post something. Probably because they would be holding up the ribbon border that frayed and tore soon after I put it up.

So yeah. I don't have such high expectations for my future workspace, but I definitely need one. Currently, I work wherever I can find a chair, my laptop perched precariously on my knees. Sometimes I score the dining room table—definitely better for my posture—or the living room couch. Most of the time, though, I sit down to work and I am distracted—by children, chores, responsibilities other than my pressing work, and life. Yes. Life distracts me.

There is something alarming in that. Camus would have a field day with it.

But my need for a desk goes beyond a place for storage and displays. Beyond a place to post reminders and stack bills. I need a desk because I need something that will be mine. My place. My drawers. My ratty bulletin board. My piles of paper that need sorting. Each time I look for a place to park my laptop and my bag, I am like a vagrant in my own home. I am constantly in someone's way and can never just find that *spot*. The one no one else can touch but me.

Stephen King once wrote about this huge mahogany desk he had. He was so proud of it that he planted it in the center of a room. And proceeded to never use it. He wound up moving it into a small corner, and he famously said:

"It starts with this: put your desk in the corner, and every time you sit down there to write, remind yourself why it isn't in the middle of the room. Life isn't a support system for art. It's the other way around."

In my case, I don't even have a desk to move to a corner. My real estate consists of whatever chair is available. And art? It's getting buried under my children's homework assignments and my own workload that piles up each week.

I need a desk. Not to stick in the middle of a room or decorate like a Christmas tree, but to escape to. I need a desk, and I need to claim it like Columbus. Stick a flag into the flat wooden surface and declare it the official space of yours truly. I've made peace with the idea that it won't be featured in Pottery Barn, but whatever desk I get, it will solely be mine. Ripped ribbon and all. Splintered wooden legs. Piles of papers and mismatched folders.

I don't have a desk, but I need one.

The Fourth Witch

I was writing a Macbeth exam for my one of my classes and I wanted to find a poem, or a song, or something that the students could relate to the text. I searched all over but couldn't find what I wanted.

So instead, I wrote what I was looking for.

I posted it on my blog and immediately started getting comments and emails about it. People were concerned. Empathetic. Some good friends laughed at the "silent" line. I took another look at the poem and saw what they noticed.

I wonder if the small bursts of inspiration that are jotted down in haste reflect larger ideas and thoughts that our conscious mind does not immediately recognize or connect to. Who is that fourth witch, the one who watches helplessly from the sidelines while Macbeth is manipulated and brought to ruin? I'm not so sure. I can analyze my own writing and try to unearth my motivations, and maybe they are profound and worthy of analysis. Sometimes the unconscious speaks louder than the conscious.

But other times? Other times the words are just a question on a Macbeth exam.

I am the fourth witch, the one they don't mention
Hidden in the shadows of the heath
While my sisters double and bubble
And secretly toil.

I am the judger, the one who observes
Watching them munch and munch
With the lives of sailors and kings
And worthy thanes.

I am the silent one, cloaked in shade
As chaos and storms brew
Nighttime cauldrons and haunted minds
And poisoned breasts.

I am the eyes of the hearer, the ears of the watcher
The witness to all that is flawed, and steeped in blood
So thick and deep and spreading
And staining.

They dance round and round, without me
The fourth sister, the banished and alone,
Cowering-in-the-corner sister.
Clean-chinned and clothed in robes
That don't quite fit.

He comes near, bold and wild,
A foul man, a fair idiot, playing upon our stage,
Fretting and strutting into their hands
And their winding charms.

"Out, Out!" I want to say. "Turn, hound!
And follow lighted tapers to a new morning

Away from these fools and their chants
And hollow knocks."

But I am the fourth witch, a role never borne
Weaker than my sisters, unsexed on the heath.
Pricking my thumb and letting him go
The way to dusty death

In silence.

How to Get Out of Bed at 5 a.m.

Believe it or not, since I announced I was training to run a half-marathon, the number-one question hasn't been, "Are you out of your f-ing mind?"

I found that a bit surprising because—and this might come as a shock to those that know me—I'm not exactly the most "fit" person out there. I thought people would assume I was kidding with this whole marathon thing and think it was some elaborate joke. Like at any moment I might yell "Color War!" and start throwing confetti and papers with team names and captains.

So shockingly, no one really questioned it. I guess they have a bit of faith in me.

Actually, the number-one question I get has to do with my training habits. Mainly the 5 a.m. training run. That's the point most of my friends have been stuck on, quickly followed by the confession of "I could never get out of bed that early."

It's true. If you had asked me a few months ago if I could get out of bed at 5 a.m., I would have laughed. I could go *to* bed at 5 a.m. But waking up? Not a chance.

So how do you wake up at 5 a.m. to run? Here's how. First, you need to really not want to see anybody. One of the perks of running at 5 a.m. is that the streets are empty, the sky is still dark, and no one's likely to see my pathetic ass running through the streets and dodging spiders. It's awesome. In fact, the random car that happens to drive by actually increases my speed. Especially if it's a van. A sketchy white van? I can sprint like the wind.

Second, did you see *Rocky*? Remember when he goes out to run and drinks the raw eggs? So, no. I'm not drinking the raw eggs, but I am definitely channeling his whole look in that scene. When I go out on my South Florida streets, I am freakin' Rocky in Philadelphia. Without the steps. Or the crowds of fans. Or, you know, his pace and leg strength. But whatever. The theme song is on my playlist.

It's also a lot easier to get up at 5 a.m. when you have no other alternative. Once I publicly announced that I was running in a half-marathon, I was pretty much screwed. I had to go through with it. There is no greater motivator than the threat of public embarrassment, and since I can rarely get out to run at night, it's 5 a.m. or nothing.

The other thing that gets me up at 5 a.m. is the whole reason I'm running in the first place. It sounds like just something you put on your fundraising page, but it's true. When you believe in what you are doing, you really can do anything. Including getting up at 5 a.m.

My 5 a.m. brain is addled and pissed off. Odds are that I was up numerous times in the night and didn't get to bed before midnight. My husband and kids are asleep when I walk out the door. Even though it looks like a cool night (morning?) outside, the temperature is hovering somewhere between eighty-five and ninety, and I'm sweating before I even leave my driveway. But even with all that, every day when I go running in my neighborhood, I am straight up thinking of the money I am raising for a cause that is so important.

And having the support of my friends—including one who said he would stand at the end of the race with a sign that says "I KNOW YOU WON'T SEE THIS ADINA BECAUSE YOU PROBABLY PASSED OUT AT MILE 3"—really spurs me on. It isn't that I'm doing this myself. I think of every person who sent me a message of encouragement. Every time I want to quit and go home, those voices play out in my head and I keep going.

Getting up at 5 a.m. definitely hovers just above one of the lower circles of hell. No question. There are days that the forces of gravity actually suck me back under my blankets, and I have to claw my way out of bed, fighting the laws of physics. There are days that I go out on the street, and even before Fort Minor starts blasting in my earbuds, I have already convinced myself that I should turn around and take a "rest day."

But I go anyway. Because the other perk of waking up at 5 a.m. to run is that no matter how bad my run is, no matter how slow my pace, no matter how many spiders I have to dodge and vans I have to outrun, at the very least, I am out there. I am trying. I am running.

I am doing something I never thought I could do.

I'm awake at 5 a.m. And for that moment, I have triumphed over my insecurities, my self-doubt, and the actual laws of physics and nature. At 5 a.m., the world is mine.

That's how I get myself out of bed.

Things I've Learned in the First Weeks of Training for a Marathon

Well, actually, a half-marathon.

You would think that running would be a natural progression from, you know, walking. It turns out that running is in a completely different world. And having gotten it into my head that I am running a half-marathon in a few months, that little tidbit took me by surprise.

The first time I went running (if you can even call it that), I was clutching my heart at the stop sign at the end of my block. I was also thanking the powers that be that it was 5:00 a.m., and no one could see me die in what was clearly the most embarrassing way possible. Realizing I needed some guidance, I bought some books with titles like *The Non-Runner's Handbook* and *The Beginner's Guide to Running* and *Get Started Running!*—all of which started with harrowing stories of people who could only run three miles.

Three miles?? I was still working on getting to the stop sign without calling 911. I had committed to running in the race, so I needed to figure out how to proceed. Because at that point, the idea of running even one mile was so laughable that I considered quietly removing myself from the marathon page and hiding out for a year under my covers. Eating chocolate. And cake.

Needless to say, getting myself to that first mile was a steep learning curve.

It's only been a few weeks since I started this insanity, and I've made my share of ridiculous rookie mistakes. But I have also learned from them.

So here is a list of the top lessons I learned from my first few weeks that I wish I had known before those tragic first days. I am sure there will be more as I progress. But there must be other people like me who were not blessed with the gazelle DNA that seems to grace the runners who post cheerfully on my newsfeed, glowing from their morning runs.

This is my paying-it-forward moment. You're welcome.

1. The spiders dangling from the trees are not as dangerous as the cars on the busy street. Flinch with caution.

2. Runderwear is a thing and it is glorious.

3. No matter how many favorite songs are on your running playlist, there will always be one that you will want to skip anyway.

4. You will develop a new understanding of measurement as it relates to driving. I now actually know what Waze means when it says, "In a half a mile, turn left."

5. Runners are the friendliest group of people you will ever meet. That runner's high thing clearly keeps them all happy. Which leads me to . . .

6. That runner's high thing is actually a thing. The first time I actually ran that mile? I was a golden goddess. No joke.

7. Bluetooth headphones. That's all.

8. Running socks are the best things to happen to socks since, well, socks.

9. Target is probably not where you want to get your

running shoes. This was a shock to me, but when I bought legit running shoes from a running store, I understood the difference, and my running world changed significantly. Target has some nice apparel. And caps. Use those. But get real shoes.

10. People run in the rain. And the snow. And finishing a run with rain on your face? Have you seen *Shawshank Redemption?* Do you remember that scene? That.

11. Running in temperatures above ninety degrees is equivalent to being in one of those dreams where you are trying to run but can't get anywhere. Unless no one else has those dreams. I'm sure that can't just be me.

12. Running at the same pace as walking is still harder than walking at the same pace as running. Take a minute to ponder that.

13. Cardiac arrest is not nearly as imminent as it might seem when you first start running. After all, I seem to have survived the daily stop-sign heart attack.

14. Nothing is more soul crushing than Facebook friends who post their workouts and ten-mile runs on a daily basis with self-serving hashtags (#IAMAWESOME!). Or the twenty-year-old who posts about her first day of training (#FIRSTDAY15MILES! #IROCK) right after you hobble in from your 3.1-mile pseudo-run. Remember that you are only competing with yourself. No one else. Feel free to borrow some of my hashtags (#SCREWYOU #MADEITTOTHESTOPSIGN #IBIRTHEDFIVEBABIESBITCH). Definitely makes the training a whole lot better.

15. Running for a cause you believe in is the single greatest motivator to get up at 5 a.m.—better than any fitness goals you might want to attain.

I Have a Meniscus! (And Other Things I Learned After Running in a Marathon)

So after nine months of training, I finally ran in the Miami Marathon. I use the term "ran" a bit liberally because in truth, it wasn't 13.1 miles of solid running as I had envisioned it. But regardless of the details, it was an extraordinary experience, made all the more meaningful by the funds I raised for an organization I care about. There are a number of things I learned while training for the event, and having gone the 13.1 miles, I now know something about actually *running* in these things. So here goes. My list of things I learned from running in a marathon (or half-marathon):

1. You don't actually start at the gun. This is something I wish I had known beforehand because I wouldn't have been so brutally honest about my expected finish time. Based on your estimated pace, they place you in different corrals. I was in corral J, which clearly stands for "Just kidding." The only comfort I got was that there was a K group behind me. In any event, group J started crossing the start line forty-five minutes after group A did. So that's a huge downer and pretty much sucks. Next time, I'm saying I can finish in an

hour. Of course, most of the people running on my team were with me in J land, so there's that.

2. There are bathrooms on the side of the road that have wait times of close to ten minutes. I stopped at one of them and watched in horror as thousands of people passed me by, knowing my race time was going to be pathetic. Afterward, some running friends told me they don't stop for the potties. They just pee on themselves as they run. I'll pause to let you think about that for a second. It made me really happy that I was not on that level of runner. I'll take the ten-minute time deficit and use the toilet. I'm good.

3. Mile 10 defies the laws of physics and time. It is straight up the longest mile ever. It's also the time to dig into those energy jelly beans that are seriously a gift from God. I don't think I ate them as much as inhaled them.

4. The best part of running a half-marathon, other than getting to the finish line, is getting to the point where the path divides between the half-marathoners and the full-marathoners. I was turning off to finish the last two miles or so when I glanced at the people who were off to run another fifteen miles, and all I could think was, "Bye, Felicia!"

5. If the weather is bad, the first three miles are harder than the last. I was ready to quit after mile 1 and was really worried. I mean, that was supposed to be the easy part! But it was pouring rain, fifty degrees, and windy, and the first part of the race was over a causeway. I wanted to die.

6. There are ways to cheat, and people actually do. I didn't, but I was tempted when I saw other people cut out a mile and a half of their run by crossing over a divider and going the other way. I could have cheated, but I was in it for the whole run. It was 13.1 miles or nothing for me. And seriously? Who are you even cheating against??

7. I really admire the people who cheer on the side of the road. I mean, what do they care if I run or not? But they definitely help move you along. I high-fived everyone I could. Best part? Seeing my brother and his wife who came out

from Jersey to cheer me along at mile 8. There is nothing like seeing family along the route.

8. At a certain point I straight up could not feel my feet. It was equal parts worrisome and awesome. If I had blisters, I would just not even know. Win!

9. Running with someone is crucial around mile 9. I met up with some people who were running on the same team, and it definitely made the whole mile 10 nightmare go a lot smoother.

10. After the race was finished, I could have eaten an entire bear. No joke. I would have ripped it apart and eaten that sucker raw. That's how hungry you are. I don't think I ever scarfed down that much food in such a short span of time.

11. Your body will want to kill you for a few days after the run. I was walking around like a ninety-year-old for a week, trying to score some cortisone shots in back alleys and abandoned buildings.

12. Crossing the finish line was kind of like giving birth. I had trained for months, went through the labor of the run, and finally crossed the finish line. It was painful. It was emotional. But it was powerful and unbelievable. And I would do it again.

Just faster.

"It's Only a 10K..."

I'm not sure when the transformation occurred, so it must have happened slowly. But a few weeks ago, when I went to Vegas to run in the Rock 'n' Roll Marathon, my friends made some comments:

"Wow! You've become an athlete!"

"I could never do that. That's amazing."

"So you're really into this running thing?"

But I stopped them, because I didn't run the Vegas marathon. Or the half. I ran the 10K. So I told them, really, it wasn't that impressive. It was only a 10K.

As soon as I said it though, I realized how ridiculous I sounded, and I wondered what had happened—what kind of space–time malfunction took place that allowed the words "It's only a 10K" to come out of my mouth. Because if you know me—if you know my relationship with exercise and healthy habits and all things green—then you also know that the idea of running a 10K (6.2 miles if you're math impaired) should never, ever, in the history of all that is "Adina Ciment" be prefaced with the phrase "it's only."

Especially since my 10K run was spectacular only in how pathetic it was. In a stunning display of agility and athletic prowess, I tripped twice. The first one was not just a little trip, by the way. This was a full-blown, flat-on-my-face, embrace-the-gods-of-gravity-and-just-go-with-it fall. Most people just ran around me or leaped over me, focused on beating their PRs (that's personal records, for those who aren't aware). Some yelled, "Are you okay?" as they soared past. I was. I got up, brushed myself off, reminded myself that as cool as the Vegas Strip looked, it would make sense to watch out for things like, you know, street curbs, and continued moving.

I tripped a second time, but didn't go down. That time, I ran a little too close to the gutter, my foot turned, and I lost my balance. I'm not sure which was more tragic—the first, all-out, pavement-hitting crash, or the second one, which must have looked like I was shoved by some invisible force while dancing the flamenco. Ever have a sputtering cough? Imagine that in human form. That was me. The only good part was that in an effort to stay balanced, I covered the few feet of chaos at my fastest pace yet.

Add to that my inability to work my running app, which decided, right as the gun went off, to switch into some mode that I had never used nor knew existed. I spent the first mile pushing buttons, trying to get back my music and my running map. I finally just shut off my phone completely, but even that took effort.

Freakin' iPhone update.

So my 10K was not that impressive, to say the least. When I crossed the finish line, I was so relieved it was only a 10K. If you're going to have a bad run, and it's going to be in front of thousands of people and photographers and ridiculously fit and toned ninety-year-olds that run faster than you, well, then, you'll be pretty thankful you didn't sign up for the half-marathon.

Still, for me to blurt out "It's only a 10K" was kind of shocking.

Maybe my problem is that even though I ran a half-marathon last year, I still don't think of myself as a serious runner. I get angry when I see people posting their runs with mile times that I know I will never hit. I get annoyed at the effort it takes for me to get out of bed to run, knowing that I will probably never regard it with anticipation. Not the way I look forward to chocolate. Or Netflix. I may think that a 10K isn't the biggest deal, but I am far from belonging to that crew of sprinters and long-legged runners who seem to glide over the pavement, leaving glitter and rainbows in their wake.

Running any distance makes the shorter distances a walk in the park. I remember when I ran my first mile—how excited I was, how proud I was. Now, that first mile is sometimes something I have to slog through in an effort to train for the longer distances, when in the beginning, that first mile *was* my longer distance. Having that one moment where the words "It's only a 10K" fell from my lips reminds me that even if I never run another race, there was a time when something that once seemed daunting became suddenly approachable.

It's somewhat symbolic. The harder life is—the longer you have to run—the easier the smaller challenges become. They are the 10Ks of our lives. Some people are still struggling through their first run, where hitting that one-mile mark is the hardest thing they have ever done. But at a certain point, you're going to run a 5K. Or a 10K. Or a half-marathon. And suddenly you're wishing for that one-mile finish line again. In that sense, "It's only a 10K" is more a statement on perspective than athletic ability.

So don't worry about me. I might have a half-marathon and two 10Ks under my belt, but it isn't going to my head. I'm still just running for a cause more than I'm trying to PR in the Miami Half-Marathon this January.

After all, it's just a half-marathon.

The Books on the Shelves

I'm cleaning out my bookshelves and getting rid of books. Marie Kondo-ing my space and deciding what sparks joy and what does not.

Okay, maybe not completely Marie Kondo style.

I don't think I can properly explain how difficult it is to do that. Over the years, and with the help of Amazon Prime, I have amassed an impressive collection of books. They're everywhere, and while I like to think that my library has some serious Beauty and the Beast potential, I also know that it's time to downsize.

Not gonna lie, I am having a hard time letting go. But I am prioritizing titles and deciding what to do with the ones that don't make the cut.

Harry Potter—the entire set, copies and all—is a keeper. The hardcover first editions that I purchased as they were released will stay on my shelf. I'm also keeping the paperback editions to lend out. And, of course, the foreign editions that I've never read but love looking at. Also the extended library. Those all stay.

Then there are the books that have been signed by various authors and, of course, all the Neil Gaiman books—signed and unsigned—that have the coveted shelf right above the Potter collection. These are easy decisions. And obviously, I'm keeping the classics: my Shakespeare collection, Dante, Camus, and a shelf of titles for a solid high-school lit curriculum (or as my son calls it, the "Shelf of books I can SparkNote").

I have children's books as well. Titles I salvaged from my parents' house that no one has ever read but me and my kids: *Good Night Veronica, Mrs. Discombobulous, Just Alike Princes, Andrew Henry's Meadow*. They are books I read with my kids that are out of print, and more than likely were never reprinted after their first run. It's easy to separate those from the ones I am not attached to: the Barbie and superhero books, the Barney books, the Teletubbies books. My kids read them and then tossed them, but for some reason, over the years, I just left them on the shelves.

Then there are others that have not been read or touched in years that I still hang on to, thinking about how one day my children will want to read them to their own children. Each of my kids has a favorite book, the one I had to read a thousand times, every night. The one they remember falling into, lost in the pictures or the words. Sometimes, it is just one picture that conjures up the memory:

"I remember that door and I wanted to jump into it."

"I loved that one picture of the dog and the birds. It was my favorite page."

There is something sacrosanct about all my books. I love seeing them on the shelves, transporting myself to when I first read them. Getting rid of them is like losing a memory, and losing the chance to hand them to a friend with the urgent plea, "Oh my God, read this!" I think about this as I take them down and put them in boxes, offering titles up for free on various WhatsApp groups, wondering what home or shelf they will find themselves on.

As I go through my bookshelves, I empty literal and figurative chapters of my life: the time when reading children's books trumped reading classics, when mindless chick lit (am I even allowed to use that term?) was my go-to, when I eschewed fiction and devoured memoirs. I take them off the shelves, one by one, putting some chapters away and keeping others as placeholders for times in my life. The ones I choose to keep—the ones written by friends, my well-worn classics, my graphic novels, my childhood picture books—are more than books to lend and share and reread. They are like tiny Pensieves, holding memories and moments that are triggered by their scent, their touch, their pictures.

It's interesting what we attach ourselves to and the meaning we ascribe to objects that somehow, over years, become important not in functionality but just in being. I may be cleaning out my bookshelves and getting rid of books, but I'm also creating a uniquely specific, finely curated home library that tells its own story. A story told not only by what is kept, but what is discarded.

An ongoing story that continues with the next Amazon delivery.

We're All Mad Here

While standing outside on a line for a port-a-potty at 5:30 a.m., I had a sudden epiphany that most runners must have some kind of undiagnosed mental illness. Put aside the whole running 13.1 or 26.2 miles, because that's not crazy enough. I'm talking about waking up at 4:30 a.m., standing in corrals until a gun goes off, and then just Forrest Gumping it on city streets with no purpose except reaching the finish line. Which you can reach with a car. Or an Uber. Or not even bother to reach and just stay sleeping like most normal people on a Sunday morning.

But for some reason, a year after I ran a half-marathon, I was back at it again, standing with thirty thousand other runners, waiting for the moment I could cross the start line and begin the long run to the finish line.

Objectively, it looks like a collection of the insane. Thousands of people in various dress—in fluffy tutus, in costumes, in skintight leggings, in sweatshirts and tank tops, in T-shirts with funny sayings and shirts with corporate logos. We gather at an ungodly hour to reenact the original

26.2 miles run by Pheidippides, which, fun fact, he wound up dropping dead from.

I know I'm not like the runners that lined up that morning. I don't really like running, and as much as I was looking forward to the finish line, I was also looking forward to not waking up to run the day after the race. Or the next day. Or the entire week. Maybe the month.

So what the hell was I doing?

Back when I first started running, I met someone at a race who asked me why I was doing it. "What is your running story?" she asked. Everyone has one. The reason they started, the reason they continue. The reason they participate in the insane gatherings of the runners.

The stories range from getting in shape, losing weight, or building stamina, to the old "bucket list," "proving you can do it," or "conquering some inner demons" reasons.

For me, running was never about conquering or anything like that. I used to joke with people who asked me how to start running by telling them that a good dose of guilt plus pain definitely helps. I had a lot of that going into my first half-marathon. I was running to raise money for an organization that helped my son and my family during a difficult time in our lives. Every training run began with thoughts of other families, and other kids, and how much I believed in the organization—and usually ended with me sobbing on the floor of my living room.

Running a race is a personal experience, but in many ways, though you're surrounded by thousands of fellow runners and people on the sidelines (who *are* those people?), it can be a somewhat lonely experience. Even with my running partners, even with the team I was running with, my experience on the course was mine alone. My throbbing ankle at mile 3, my pulled back at mile 7, my constant desire to collapse and get carried off the course like the seasoned athletes I saw at the finish line. I fought through each mile and shut down the negative mind-speak that plagued the run. And if I had to think about the insanity of what I was doing, I only had to remind myself of why I started. Back to the pain and the guilt. Back to that first mile I completed. Back to the day I learned the difference between Nike and Brooks and the value of good underwear.

Running is a celebration of all we can overcome. Each runner carries the scars and wounds that brought them there on race day: their original running story, their original reason for pushing themselves. Out there, even though we are "racing," we are pushing together—regardless of the loneliness we might feel in our minds. Yes, a fight almost broke out over the port-a-potty line. Yes, I was scarfing down caffeinated jelly beans like a junkie at mile 10. Yes, I continue to question my sanity as I lace up at 5:30 a.m. to train again for another race.

And yes, to an outsider, those runners responsible for shutting down the city streets on a major race day might look like a bizarre collection of people from some insane alternate universe.

But those T-shirts and tutus tell a visual story that only an outsider can miss: a story of goodness, of community, of strength, of drive, and of passion. Sometimes a story of guilt and pain.

But always a story of heart.

Bumper Sticker Fandom

Yesterday, someone cut in front of me on the highway. I slammed on my brakes and leaned on my horn, but the driver sped away without even a glance in his mirror. He could have waved, or, you know, signaled. But no. He was just like, "%$#@ that!" I know I shouldn't be surprised—this kind of thing happens every day—but for years I have felt there is a certain camaraderie that develops among the drivers and passengers on highways. It's in the nods and polite waves as we weave in and out of traffic or pass the slower vehicles on the road. It's in the eye-rolls when there's heavy traffic, the brief meeting of the minds when attempting to merge. The subtle "please let me in" and the silent nod of "no problem, I won't smash into you." There's the carefully averted eyes of the jerk that speeds up, the clueless driver who drifts as he's texting, and the embarrassed look after a loud horn blows him off the road.

It's a small, short-lived traveling community.

And then there is the singular bond formed with a bumper sticker.

I've seen this happen.

Back in the day, when I was sporting a "Harry for President" bumper sticker, I developed highway friends who would honk their horns and point to the Gryffindor stickers on their hatchbacks. The experience connected me to other Harry Potter fans who wished they were apparating instead of sitting in I-95 traffic.

As my fandoms changed, so did my stickers. I went through my Sherlock phase (the Benedict Cumberbatch kind), with the nondescript "221 Baker Street" magnet. My "Mother of Dragons" from *Game of Thrones* joined the crew, along with the Deathly Hallows, Appa (if you don't know, you should remedy that), and my late-to-the-party Tardis. Putting them on the back of my car was a call to others on the road to make a connection and give a salute from the next lane, acknowledging that we have read the same novels or watched the same shows. It was a call to understand—in a way that only fans can—the importance of that experience on a crowded highway.

When I started running, I sported the requisite distance magnets: 13.1, 10K, 5K, and the always funny 13.7 (I Got Lost). Placing those on my car put me in a new league of commuters—the ones who would rather be sprinting to work than sitting in a leather-upholstered front seat listening to SiriusXM. Though I was hardly a sprinter, those little signs that followed me in my car were portable medals, the not-so-subtle bragging of my accomplishments. They made me part of an elite group who knew the racing codes and the meaning behind the numbers on my tailgate.

I've seen fewer fandom stickers these past years. I guess when politics divided the country and Covid separated everyone further, the fandom stickers gave way to political affiliations and presidential candidates. Those bumper stickers form a very different society on the road, their own little community of angry "%$#@ Biden" or "%$#@ Trump" announcers, stirring up vitriol and road rage. Meanwhile, the poor "Coexist" people use their car for virtue signaling and toxic positivity. It's an interesting dynamic to watch.

Maybe the answer to the anger and divisiveness that's plaguing the country is to go back to our fandoms. We all have different destinations on the highways and roads, but if we can find commonality in a lightsaber, a dragon, or a Sorting Hat, maybe, for that one moment, we can forget our differences. Maybe we can all just sit down and kill each other with ten-sided dice.

Granted, it's easy to wax poetic about solving world problems over a DND game or a cosplay meetup and ignore the unfortunate truth that even those sacred spaces have been tainted by politics and division.

I recently had a minor fender bender and had to take my car to the shop. When I got it back, all my magnets and stickers were gone. I haven't replaced them, and so now, when I head down I-95, I'm like everyone else: angry at the traffic, barely listening to SiriusXM or the podcast I loaded, mindlessly moving forward. But I still keep an eye out for the fandom family that cuts in front of me with a Ravenclaw crest on their back windshield or a sticker with a sharp reminder of "What do we say to the god of death?"

After all, even if I'm not actively wearing the colors, we are still part of the same team. So I do what I always do: nod and wave to my fellow fan.

And then lean on my horn.

Because %$#@ that.

A Song for Miriam

I went to the ocean to sing a song for Miriam, stood looking out onto the waves as they crashed to the shore and thought about my friend. How she would have loved to have been here.

The ocean was her home, the place she went to for peace and tranquility. She shepherded men and women to the shore for healing and rejuvenation. I never joined her, promising myself that the next time, the next week, I would join her sand tribe on the beach.

And now it is too late.

This is a song for Miriam, like the Miriam of old who sang at the shore of the Red Sea with joy and celebration, leading the women who followed her to embrace the joy, to recover from trauma, to find their strength. And this Miriam, my Miriam, did the same: running to celebrations of friends and families, remaining present for those she cared for, always reminding us to embrace life. Embrace happiness. Remain authentic. She was the woman who celebrated not just a birthday, but the entire month of her birth, by traveling and experiencing the world. She was a beacon of energy, a conduit that didn't stop until, in one monstrous moment, God took her away. Suddenly and sharply.

And now, the world is colder. Is darker.

This is a song for Miriam, composed on ancient stones overlooking the Mediterranean, miles away from my Miriam. Miles away from the woman who was my confidante. My voice of reason. My friend who would sit in my living room, laughing and talking and dragging me outside to sit in the sun. Or to take a walk. I usually would say no, despite her insistence, but sometimes she would win, and I would grab my shoes. Join her at a class. Or just talk.

And now those walks have ended. Our conversations left unfinished. And now she will not visit me anymore.

This is a song for Miriam, a woman whose sudden and painful death is reverberating through my home, my community, and the world, echoing off these ancient stones where I stand above the Mediterranean, miles away, searing the loss into my soul. I weep at the water's edge, yearning with all my soul to hear the song of my Miriam. To see her on the sand. To hug her again. To take another picture.

There are no more pictures to take.

I came to the ocean to sing to her what I thought would be a mournful, tragic, painful song of loss and shock over how someone with such vitality can somehow just disappear in an instant. But as I stand by the ocean, I hear her voice in the waves, reminding me of what she always preached on multicolored status updates that inspired thousands. The call to live. To embrace life. And in a painful irony, her death has become the strongest post of all, a powerful coda to all that she tried to impart about the tenuous nature of life to those of us left behind. A reminder to go to the figurative shores of our lives, playing tambourines and dancing, and write our song of the sea. Write the song of our lives.

This is my song for my Miriam.

The Return

The holiday of Rosh Hashanah is right around the corner, and it kicks off a period of introspection and *teshuva*—a word that describes repentance but is literally translated as "return." We are supposed to look back at the choices and mistakes we have made over the past year and apologize, express contrition, and ask for the slate to be wiped clean. In essence, returning us to what we were before the sins or mistakes.

It reminds me of a theme in classical Greek literature: *nostos*, or "the return." The hero needs to come back to his home, to be celebrated for the trials and tribulations he experienced since leaving the familiar places of his youth and upbringing.

In many ways, I think everyone has a hero's journey that takes them through the same stages as the Greek heroes of the past. But sometimes the journey home is fraught with obstacles, and not everyone survives the trip. Sometimes we die on the mountain, or we get stuck on Circe's island. Maybe we forget all callings of home, happy to drift in dreams on the shores of the lotus eaters.

I've been thinking about this *nostos* recently, and not because I just finished reading *Circe* by Madeline Miller. For the past two years, the overwhelming cry in the streets has been about getting back to normal. A return to the way things were. There are different types of people when it comes to this wish: the ones who swear we will never return, the ones who ran away to find a new life, and the ones who are holding out for a tomorrow that looks like yesterday.

I'm familiar with all those types. The return is something we hope for, but it is ultimately a denial of the reality of life. I remember when my oldest child left for college. I remarked to my husband that the dynamic in the home permanently changed the day we dropped her off at the airport. As each child left to follow suit, the change became more pronounced. And though I relished the moments when they all returned home for a weekend or during a break, it was never the same as having everyone growing slowly, or quickly, under the same roof. That doesn't make it a bad thing. It's just new. It's different.

The place we return to is never the same as the place we left from. So much happens in between. Odysseus, after fighting in the Trojan War, struggles to return to Ithaca, but he can't return unchanged to his wife, Penelope, after so many years of trying to get back to what he left. The scars of battle and the trauma of his travels have forever changed him. The return to Ithaca at the end of the story is just another step in his journey, not the end of it.

I have been on many journeys.

While these journeys create strength and are catalysts for growth and change, anyone who has ventured forth still wants the return, despite knowing the difficulty of trying to get home again. And that return is often a lonely experience. Just ask Odysseus.

Perhaps it isn't about a return to normal, then. It seems the *nostos* is more geographic than emotional. Part of a hero's journey is about returning different, with something to share.

Triumphant, maybe. Or damaged. Jacob can battle with an angel and be victorious, but he will still forever limp. We return with scars and defenses, with eyes that have seen the cyclops and lips that have tasted the lotus. The message of real *teshuva*, of real return, is understanding that change. You can't just apologize and make it all good with your friends. You must be different. That is how you grow. Not a hero's return in the classic sense, but a return nonetheless.

Wishing for a return to the past may be futile, but it isn't necessarily depressing. Change, even through fire, makes us walk differently. Changes what we love. Sometimes even changes *who* we love. Contentment comes, I guess, in the knowledge that we may not be able to go back, but, like the heroes of old, we can return. We can do *teshuva*.

And that is where we begin again.

AFTERWORD

I read *Wasn't Expecting This*, in one way or another, twice. Once, as the posts went live on my mother's blog as a teenager. And more recently, for the second time in the process of this book becoming published. This time, I'm an adult. And I'm seeing that story through completely different eyes.

When you're a kid, your parents don't exist outside the identity of mom or dad. Their "before" lives are bedtime stories and photo albums. We rarely, if ever, consider the possibility that before we arrived, our parents were perhaps a little bit like us, navigating life with their own hopes and dreams, blind to the challenges that lay in wait. As I manage new changes in my own life in my late twenties, only now has this become so clear to me. Only now do I look back and wonder how the heck my mom navigated five kids, a full-time job, and everything else that was thrown at our family, doing it all without messing any of us up (that badly).

Not to mention the regular trips to Disney, arts and crafts activities, music lessons, three course shabbat meals, and directing a musical just so I could finally be in a school production. In other words, everything that made growing up in my house special.

In all truth, I don't think it's fair to say I really lived the story that's told in these pages. Because I didn't. I was a teenager when most of these events took place and I never fully saw the impact that they had on my mom and the rest of my family. Granted, I was the oldest kid. An oldest daughter. So I was somewhat in tune with family happenings in an elevated way. But I was still a kid who would never — could never — understand certain things. Like what a double mastectomy can do to someone's experience of womanhood, or what it's like to watch your child get diagnosed with a brain tumor. I knew the other perspective: seeing a mother who can't cook dinner after her surgery. My little brother lying motionless on the couch and me thinking he's trying to make a joke. And the aftermath of all of that.

I can't remember a specific time my mother sat me down to break some terrible news to me. She has a knack for keeping us all in the loop, but softening the blows, often with sarcasm, dark humor and an arsenal of positive statistics. There was never a bombshell moment. I knew that cancer was involved, but there was never a definitive "I have cancer" declaration. We knew my brother had a brain tumor, but it was benign and he would probably be fine. We were all going to be fine. And I wholeheartedly believed it.

I never considered what it might have taken for my mother to arm herself with this optimism. I never considered the sleepless nights of doom-scrolling on reddit in search of that one factoid that rings of hope.

The fear, anguish, and anger in these pages is something I, as her daughter, rarely got to see in action. Still, things were not easy. We all still cry and comfort each other on this journey that seems to have no end. This book is perhaps the most unfiltered version of that story. Reading it now, my older self is grateful for her thorough documentation. And I am humbled to come from such strength.

I like to think that strength lives inside me too, somewhere, tucked away with all the other things I've inherited from my mother: a love for Harry Potter, Stephen King, musical theater fails and Indiana Jones. The need to write when my emotions demand it — and the ability to overcome imposter syndrome when I do.

They say a kid's worst nightmare is turning into her parents. For me, growing up is realizing I'd be lucky to.

Shoshy Ciment

ACKNOWLEDGMENTS

There are many things I never expected.

I never expected to write a non-fiction book. In fact, I never even voluntarily read non-fiction until a few years ago. But while most of my literary aspirations revolved around fantasy and magic, the people who brought me to the point of publishing are very real and very non-fiction. So it makes sense that they're making an appearance at the end of this work.

Michael Jenet, at The Journey Institute Press, has been a guiding light in this whole process. I read what to expect when publishing a book, but the care and guidance that my publisher led me with ran contrary to everything I was told. It's probably cliche to call him a prince, but I can't think of a more appropriate term. He and Dafna are the reasons this book is in your hands.

My sister, Yaffa, who I know is not expecting this, taught me everything about strength and resilience. She was also a major inspiration for my writing pursuits. Though I will always be in her shadow, it's an impressive shadow to occupy. I'm so grateful to have "the voice of Yaffa" in my life.

My friend Miriam Amselem had encouraged me to publish my essays, and I told her no one would be interested. I never expected her to pass away so suddenly but I know that wherever she is, she is smiling. I hear her loud "I told you so!" echoing daily.

The countless support people who have framed my family's last 10 years helped me put words to emotions whenever

I would call distraught, angry, or stupidly happy. Specifically, my cousin Danny Reich, Shera Dubitsky from Sharsheret, Tzvi Haber, from imadi, Moshe Turk from Team Lifeline, Ahuva Orlofsky, and Gila Pfeffer whose story on a random Sharsheret video literally saved my life and whose humor has sustained it since. Additionally, the organizations who held our hands through a difficult few years: Sharsheret, Chai Lifeline, the Ohr Meir Foundation, Rofeh Cholim Cancer Society, and the Pediatric Low Grade Glioma Foundation. Special shout-out to the small community of brain tumor parents on Facebook who answer questions faster than I can refresh MyChart.

Finally, a thank you to my kids who have to put up with me as their mom; each of you carries yourself with the grace and resilience I wish I had and have exceeded any expectations. And Avi: You took my essays and put them together into a book as a gift for me so that I could see what it was like to be a writer. Because of you, I sent out queries. Because of you, we survived so much of what we never expected.

I don't know what to expect next, but I will no doubt be meeting it with you.

ABOUT THE AUTHOR

Adina Ciment is a writer and educator from South Florida where she lives with her husband and five children. After teaching High School English for 30 years, she started The Raven Writing Company, a private tutoring company. Her essays have appeared on HuffPost, Kveller, Tailslate, and Aish.Com and she has been a keynote speaker for various non-profit organizations. Wasn't Expecting This is her first book.

Journey Institute Press

Journey Institute Press is a non-profit publishing house created by authors to flip the publishing model for new authors. Created with intention and purpose to provide the highest quality publishing resources available to authors whose stories might otherwise not be told.

JI Press focusses on women, BIPOC, and LGBTQ+ authors without regard to the genre of their work.

As a Publishing House, our goal is to create a supportive, nurturing, and encouraging environment that puts the author above the publisher in the publishing model.

Storytellers Publishing is an Imprint of Journey Institute Press, a division of 50 in 52 Journey, Inc.

THE
JOURNEY P
INSTITUTE
P R E S S